Ultimate Beauty 2024

#1 Face and Skin

Creator: Reed, Elizabeth M., author.

Title: Ultimate beauty 2024: #1 face and skin / Elizabeth M. Reed.
ISBN: 9781923212107 (paperback)
Series: Ultimate beauty ; 1
Notes: Includes index.

Subjects: Face--Care and hygiene.
Skin--Care and hygiene.
Cosmetics.
Beauty, Personal.

Dewey Number: 646.726

Leaves of Gold Press

ABN 67 099 575 078
PO Box 345, Shoreham, 3916, Victoria, Australia
www.leavesofgoldpress.com

Ultimate Beauty 2024

#1 Face and Skin

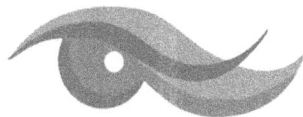

Elizabeth M. Reed, B.A. (Hons) Dip. Ed.

Other books in this series:

Ultimate Beauty #2 2024

Hair, Body & Smile

Elizabeth M. Reed, B.A. (Hons) Dip. Ed.

CONTENTS

PART 5: HOME-MADE SKIN CARE RECIPES

Legend

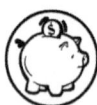

Frugal: Economical ways of achieving cosmetic improvements.

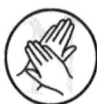

Non-surgical: Cosmetic techniques in which no instruments penetrate the skin.

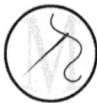

Minimally-invasive: Cosmetic techniques that involve minor incisions with surgical instruments but usually require no general anesthesia.

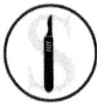

Surgical: Cosmetic techniques that involve an incision with surgical instruments.

FOREWORD

Most of us want to look our best, just like all those 'ageless' movie stars. Finding the perfect cosmetic treatment, however, can be confusing. What treatments are available? Which of them best suits your needs and budget?

Hunting down all your options, finding conveniently located salons or clinics and reading reviews from other clients all takes time.

For your convenience, the 'Beauty' series of books helps to solve the problem. We make the job of finding the appropriate cosmetic treatments quick and easy, for both men and women. Dozens of beauty techniques have been described and compared for you, so that you can find the most suitable therapy available.

THE EASY GUIDE TO CHOOSING

It is sometimes difficult to find information about ways to improve your appearance. Every day, thousands of people are having cosmetic enhancements, but most of them prefer to keep that fact secret, and avoid talking about it.

In this series 'Ultimate Beauty Books 1 & 2', we compare the latest cosmetic treatments, techniques and procedures.

The aim is to provide you with the convenience of comparison and the benefit of explanatory articles.

Armed with this information, you will be in the best position to evaluate your cosmetic treatment requirements.

This enables you to avoid spending your time calling or visiting numerous salons and clinics to compare treatments and products with often-confusing brand names. It also helps you find a treatment or product better suited to your needs, at a given price point.

RETURN TO THE 'YOU' YOU KNEW

People have been enhancing their looks with potions, lotions, plucking, shaving, dyes, powders, paints, tattoos, corsets, wigs, jewelry and so on since the dawn of the human race. In the 21st century, more sophisticated cosmetic treatments are undergoing a surge of popularity throughout the world.

There are many reasons why people seek cosmetic treatments. Skin blemishes such as acne, eczema, spider veins and rosacea can cause people to feel uncomfortable in social situations. Excess hair on the face or body can be embarrassing, too. As we age, our skin loses elasticity and may sustain sun damage, leading to wrinkles, pigmentation and sagging. Dieting alone may not remove fat deposits from certain areas of the body, such as the hips, belly or upper arms. This is where techniques such as liposuction or non-invasive fat treatments may be useful.

We all want to look our best, and these days there are many safe, quick rejuvenating and skin tightening therapies available.

Numerous appearance-enhancement techniques are now being offered. The range of choices might surprise you – for instance, many people might think that loss of eyebrow hair cannot be redressed; however there is even a way of making eyebrows appear thick again, and shaping them to flatter your face. Another procedure, cosmetic tattooing, is a way of applying semi-permanent makeup, so that you don't have to apply eyeliner or mascara every day. There are even non-surgical treatments for patchy baldness.

More and more non-surgical cosmetic techniques are now being offered. It is no longer necessary to 'go under the knife' to achieve improvements.

COMPARE COSMETIC TREATMENTS.

When – or if – you decide you are ready to rejuvenate your appearance with something more than over-the-counter or home-made cosmetic treatments, where do you start to look? There is an enormous and bewildering array of possibilities offered by an ever-burgeoning number of clinics and salons. Which technique is best for your particular needs?

That is the question these books aim to answer. They provide you with the information needed to compare cosmetic treatments so that you can make an educated choice.

In describing these treatments, all efforts have been made to be objective and unbiased. A broad description of each technique is given, without much elaboration on details.

These books do not recommend any particular cosmetic treatments and it is up to the consumer to consult their practitioner on associated topics such as psychological issues, pre- and post-treatment protocols, contraindications, side-effects, potential risks and complications, price and possible discomfort.

Welcome to these pages. Enjoy browsing!

Elizabeth M. Reed

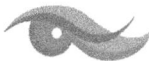

Search for cruelty-free cosmetics online. Scan this QR code with any scanning app on your phone or other device.

Cruelty-Free
Beauty Products

We recommend that you always choose to buy cruelty-free beauty products. They can be identified by this symbol.

Testing products on animals is not merely a matter of dabbing some nail polish on a rabbit's claws, or wiping some shampoo on a beagle's ears. I will not distress readers by describing exactly how beauty products are tested on animals. Suffice to say that animal testing laboratories are torture chambers where horrific practices are carried out. If you wish, you can find out more here.

www.peta.org/issues/animals-used-for-experimentation/
Seek cruelty-free cosmetics here:
features.peta.org/cruelty-free-company-search/index.aspx

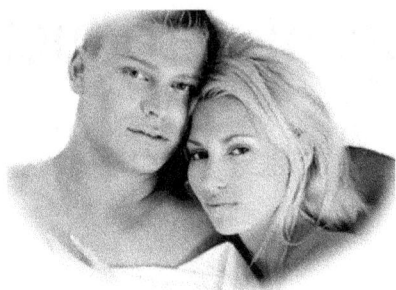

INTRODUCTION

PERSONAL BEAUTY

The esteem and pursuit of personal beauty is as old as the human race. The first definite archeological records of makeup use come from Ancient Egyptian and Sumerian tombs dating as far back as around 3500 BC. These people used soot and other natural ingredients to paint their faces and bodies, and even manufactured special tools to apply their makeup. In South Africa, archaeological sites provide evidence that people may have used body paint more than 50,000 years ago, indicating that they painted their bodies before they even wore clothes. Even our nearest relatives, the Neanderthals, may have worn makeup and jewelry to enhance their personal beauty.

WHY DO WE WANT TO LOOK GOOD?

Most men and women would say that when they look good they feel good. Scientists tell us that human beings are 'hard-wired' to be attracted to good-looking people. Feeling attractive to others can boost our self-esteem.

Human beings are social animals and by our very nature, it is essential to us to feel accepted and loved; even admired. All in all, life generally seems better when you look your best.

Looking good may make you appear not only more desirable, but also cleverer and more virtuous. In many cases, humans attribute positive characteristics, such as intelligence and honesty, to physically attractive people without consciously realizing it.[1]

From research done in the United States and United Kingdom, it was found that the association between intelligence and physical attractiveness is stronger among men than among women.[2]

WHAT MAKES A FACE ATTRACTIVE?

Beauty is said to be 'in the eye of the beholder'. But why exactly do you find certain faces attractive? Is it well-defined features, clear skin, wide eyes? Research has shown that we can identify the elements of 'beauty'.

Why do we consider these elements to be beautiful? Because of human evolution. At a primal level, human beings are 'programmed' to seek a healthy mate. A healthy mate will possess good genes to pass on to their children, and the facial elements we perceive as beautiful or handsome can signify good genes.

Symmetry

To the human eye, the ideal beautiful female or handsome male face must be close to symmetrical. In 2009, a research team from Osaka University tried to discover the most important factors for facial beauty. Their conclusion – a perfectly beautiful face required both symmetry and 'averageness'. The theory is based on our instinctive desire for survival as a species. When choosing a partner to have children with, our natural (often unconscious) inclination is to choose a healthy person. A fit and healthy partner is more likely to have 'good

---

1   Dion K, Berscheid E, Walster E (December 1972). "What is beautiful is good". J Pers Soc Psychol 24 (3): 285–90. doi:10.1037/h0033731. PMID 4655540.

2   Kanazawa Satoshi (2011). "Intelligence and physical attractiveness". Intelligence 39 (1): 7–14. doi:10.1016/j.intell.2010.11.003

genes' and will therefore be more likely to produce and raise healthy children.[3]

But does a symmetrical face really indicate a healthy body? This controversial theory actually has a wealth of evidence to back it up. Australian psychologist Gillian Rhodes co-authored a ground-breaking study that compared facial symmetry with medical records. She discovered that the most beautiful faces actually belonged to people with the best health. 'This preference for symmetry,' she wrote, 'may be biologically based.'[4]

"Symmetry works because the idea is that if you have a history of poor developmental stability—for example, a major illness or a nutrition deficiency early on—then you tend to have asymmetrical features," researcher Dr. Viren Swami explains. Thus, evolutionary psychologists believe humans have 'evolved to find healthy facial features attractive, and symmetrical facial features are a good indication of health.'[5]

Unremarkableness or averageness

Why do we feel attracted to 'average' or 'unremarkable' faces? The Osaka team found that on some basic and subconscious level, when we see an unusual face we are hard-wired to view the man or woman as 'unhealthy', and therefore less attractive. This inbuilt prejudice appears to be common to all human beings, regardless of culture, race or religion.

Smooth skin and even skin color

It's not just symmetry and averageness that make faces attractive. A luminous, unblemished complexion is another factor. Smooth,

---

3   *Effect of averageness and sexual dimorphism on the judgment of facial attractiveness. Masashi Komoria, Satoru Kawamurab, Shigekazu Ishiharac, DOI: 10.1016/j.visres.2009.03.005*

4   *Facial symmetry and the perception of beauty. Gillian Rhodes and Fiona Proffitt, Jonathan M. Grady and Alex Sumich. Psychonomic Bulletin & Review 1998, 5 (4), 659-669*

5   *Swami, V., and Furnham, A. (2008). The Psychology of physical attraction. London: Routledge.*

evenly-colored skin in both sexes gives the impression of youth and good health. Conversely blotches, discolored patches, blemishes and lesions signal poor health or aging. This is why foundation and cover-up makeup play a big part in making women look more attractive.

'Both skin topography (smoothness or bumpiness) and skin coloration affect the perception of facial age, health and attractiveness,' says researcher B. Fink. 'Skin topography seems to be a strong age cue while skin coloration is a stronger predictor of facial health perception.'

When we're young and healthy, our skin is flawless. But as we get older, our skin tends to discolor and lose its smooth texture, whether from sun-damage, scars or other kinds of injury. It is no surprise that concealing such imperfections makes us look younger and healthier.

Consciously or not, we all use skin appearance to make judgments about a person's health. In the study cited, researchers cropped photographs of cheek skin from 170 women and girls, aged 11 to 76. They asked 353 men and women to rate each cheek sample for attractiveness, health and youth. They also asked them to guess (based on nothing more than a cheek image) the age of the person in the photograph.[6]

Raters' guesses about the ages of the subjects tended to be accurate. The older the subject of the photograph, the less likely they were to be rated healthy, attractive and youthful. Nonetheless, one factor defeated age: The skin samples with even tone and texture were rated as younger, healthier and more attractive. Smooth, even skin tone and texture are signs of good health and minimal sun damage. No wonder human beings find it attractive.

For the survival of the species human beings are 'wired' to see skin free from acne, pigmentation disorders or other dermatological issues as indicating healthy genes, and hence better chances of begetting healthy offspring.

---

6   *Color homogeneity and visual perception of age, health, and attractiveness of female facial skin. P. J. Matts, B. Fink, K. Grammer and M. Burquest. Journal of the American Academy of Dermatology, Vol. 57, pp.977-984, 2007*

The good news is, you have some control over this issue. Your diet and lifestyle play a more vital role in your skin's appearance than even your genetic inheritance. If you want to have even skin-tone, wear sunscreen. Most uneven skin color is caused by sun damage. Daily application of sunblock (preferably a zinc oxide formula) is your best protection. For an extra boost to your skin-tone, choose foods containing carotenoids, such as carrots, sweet potatoes, spinach, kale, collard greens and tomatoes.

Color in women's faces

In the animal world, females proclaim their sexual availability and reproductive quality to potential mates via physical signals and color changes. In chimpanzees for example, the female's rump turns bright red to announce her receptivity and fertility. In contrast, humans have what is often referred to as concealed ovulation, meaning that not only is it not visible, but that the woman herself is not usually aware of exactly when she ovulates. It is almost impossible to tell when a woman is fertile. Almost, but not quite impossible – there *are* subtle signs.

Examine the use of makeup across cultures and eras, and you will find a pattern. It is possible to paint color anywhere on the face; blue on the cheeks, for instance, or green on the lips. Nonetheless, all cultures, uninfluenced by each other, have concurred on certain fundamental truths about feminine beauty. In all human societies makeup is used to even out the tone of the complexion, darken the eyes, make the cheeks pinker and redden the lips. This hold as true for Japanese Geishas and Ancient Egyptians as for modern women of the Western world readying themselves for a night out.

Research indicates that women's faces are more attractive (to both sexes) closer to the time of ovulation, when they're most fertile. During this fertile period levels of the hormone estrogen rise, relative to progesterone. The hormonal alteration intensifies the flow of blood just beneath the surface of the skin. This leads to rosier cheeks and redder lips. Thus, by rouging their cheeks and applying reddening lipstick, women are accentuating their natural signs of fertility. Those red lips and pink cheeks are not only implying that the woman's body is ready to have a baby. Blood flow also increased when humans are sexually aroused; therefore that bright facial color is bound to attract the notice of potential suitors.

Color in men's faces

Color is just as vital for men's facial attractiveness, though in a different way. Recent research indicates that masculine facial features are not as important to attractiveness as skin tone. Women preferred men with yellower and redder skin tones, both of which can signal good health; an essential factor in choosing a mate. By contrast, pale, dull skin with blemishes or lesions was usually considered unattractive. Perhaps this is because such traits betray a weak immune system, according to study co-author Ian Penton-Voak, an experimental psychologist at the University of Bristol in the U.K. Instead of looking for a manly man, Penton-Voak noted, a woman may be focusing more on an immediate question: Is this potential mate healthy or sick?

Testosterone has also been shown to darken skin color, in laboratory experiments.

Contrast

Eye makeup and lipstick work together to make a face appear more feminine. 'Women tend to be naturally darker around their eyes and mouths than men of the same skin tone. When women use cosmetics to darken the eyes and lips, they are exaggerating this sex difference to make the face appear more feminine,' explains Dr. Richard Russell, an Assistant Professor of Psychology at Gettysburg College.[7]

It's the *contrast* that's important. The darker the facial features as compared to the skin tone, the more feminine a face appears. Russell's research has shown that this effect is so vital in distinguishing gender that people can perceive the same face as either male or female according to the amount of contrast.

---

7   *Aspects of Facial Contrast Decrease with Age and Are Cues for Age Perception. Aurélie Porcheron, Emmanuelle Mauger, Richard Russell. Published: March 06, 2013. DOI: 10.1371/journal.pone.0057985*

Russell also found that when the eyes or the lips of a woman's face are darkened, it becomes more attractive. The opposite is true for a man's face.

Sexual dimorphism

To some degree humans are 'programmed' to be more attracted to certain faces than others. Sexual dimorphism, meaning sex-specific characteristics, is one of the major factors in determining what we find beautiful.

Women: The more feminine a woman's features are, the more attractive she's perceived to be. 'For women, things like large eyes, a small nose and fuller lips are generally found to be more attractive since they are considered to enhance facial femininity,' says Dr. Viren Swami, a Reader in Psychology at the University of Westminster, co-author of 'The Psychology of Physical Attraction'. One study found that a bigger forehead and smaller-than-average chin and nose are seen to be more desirable in a woman. Researchers believe that we've evolved to view female-specific traits as indications of a high estrogen-to-testosterone ratio. This implies high fertility. At a fundamental level, beauty is all about producing healthy children.

Men: What about masculine facial traits? Scientific studies suggest that women, on average, tend to be attracted to men who not only display a high degree of facial symmetry but also have masculine facial characteristics such as a broad forehead, relatively longer lower face, prominent chin and brow, thin lips, chiseled jaw and defined cheekbones.[8]

---

8   *Little, A.C., Cohen, D.L., Jones, B.C., & Belsky, J. (2007). Human preferences for facial masculinity change with relationship type and environmental harshness. Behavioral Ecology and Sociobiology, 61,967–973.*

Facial hair

In women, smooth and relatively hairless facial skin indicates low levels of androgens and high estrogen. Both indicate fertility – and therefore attractiveness. This applies to the lower part of the face, not to the eyebrows and eyelashes. In healthy young women (and men), eyebrows and lashes are thick and luxuriant.

As for facial hair in men – according to one study, women and men find facial hair most attractive when it is rare in the social environment. When shown men's faces, men and women study participants consistently rated the faces with beards or stubble as more attractive than clean-shaven faces. But beards were most alluring at times when facial hair was rare, whereas clean-shaven faces gained in popularity during periods when hairy faces were the norm.[9]

Hair on the head

The scalp-hair frames the face. Given the choice, most people would prefer to have a full head of thick hair than otherwise. Abundant hair on the head is associated with youthfulness. Fortunately there are new treatments available for patchy baldness and pattern balding.

Another study indicates men who choose to go bald by shaving their heads are perceived as being more masculine, even taller and physically stronger — although less attractive than men with a full head of hair. The study was published in the peer-reviewed journal *Social Psychological & Personality Science*.

'I'm not recommending that men with thick full heads of hair shave their heads, because even if they gain in terms of dominance, they lose in terms of attractiveness,' said Albert Mannes, a lecturer at the Wharton School of Business at the University of Pennsylvania who conducted the study, 'but if you're balding, you might want to just finish what mother nature started and take it all off. You might be surprised by the positive effects.'

---

9   *Zinnia J. Janif, Robert C. Brooks and Barnaby J. Dixson. Negative frequency-dependent preferences and variation in male facial hair Biol. Lett.. 2014 10 4 20130958; doi:10.1098/rsbl.2013.0958 (published 16 April 2014) 1744-957X*

Fat distribution

Not all thin or angular faces are considered attractive. From an evolutionary viewpoint, fuller faces indicate heart health and immunity to infections. A St. Andrews University study shows that men rated 'facial adiposity' in women, (the perception of plumpness in the face), as more attractive. From an evolutionary standpoint, fuller faces indicate good heart health and a strong immune system. A healthy mother means healthy babies, which benefits human survival.

The overall look of the face

Just because you don't resemble a movie star doesn't mean you're not good-looking. It's important to remember that your *overall face* is more important to your appearance than your specific features. In other words, as long as a woman's features collectively feminize her face (even if she has a larger nose or thinner lips, for instance), she is still considered pretty. 'If high cheekbones contribute to greater femininity, then the total look would be perceived to be attractive,' Dr Swami explained, 'not necessarily just the high cheekbones on their own.'

The same applies to men, regarding masculine traits.

WHY DO PEOPLE WEAR MAKEUP?

People wear makeup for a variety of reasons, including:

- To enhance their natural beauty.
- To be more alluring.
- To boost their confidence.
- To conceal blemishes such as dark circles under the eye, age spots, pigmentation, visible pores, uneven coloring, pimples and scars.
- To 'brighten' the facial skin.
- To look younger.
- To look older (teenagers).

Actors wear makeup to counteract the washing-out effect of studio or stage lights, and clowns wear makeup as a form of disguise.

We have already touched on the question of why painting the face with makeup as an aspect of personal grooming makes people— especially women—look more attractive.

'The maintenance of youthful features and the exaggeration of female typical traits can be found in almost every culture,' says Dr. Bernhard Fink, a professor at the University of Göttingen who studies the evolutionary psychology of human mate preferences. Makeup works for women because it exaggerates (or invents) the natural signs of human youth, fertility and sexual availability, thus making them seem more appealing on an evolutionary level.[10]

Makeup has the power to change our appearance. 'Foundation smooths the skin, making it appear healthier and younger,' says Dr. Pamela Pallett, a researcher at Dartmouth University. 'Eye makeup and lipstick can also accentuate your natural femininity.' The darker and more contrasting your lips are from the surrounding skin, the more attractive.

The ancient Egyptians regarded beauty as a sign of holiness. Everything the ancient Egyptians used had a spiritual aspect to it, including cosmetics, which is why cosmetics were an integral part of their daily lives. In tombs, cosmetic palettes were found buried with the deceased as grave goods which further emphasized the idea that cosmetics were not only used for aesthetic purposes but rather magical and religious purposes.

---

10   *Facial, Olfactory, and Vocal Cues to Female Reproductive Value. Susanne Röder, Bernhard Fink, Benedict C. Jones. Evolutionary Psychology 11(2): 392-404*

Nonetheless women will often state that their male partner tells them they look prettier without makeup. It is indeed true that when men are polled about their makeup preferences, as many as one in five says that their significant other wears far too much makeup, while one in ten wishes that women did not wear makeup at all. There is no doubt that a large proportion of men will say women look prettier without it.

While that's certainly a laudable sentiment, it may not reflect the true situation. Study after study has found that when shown pictures of women with and without makeup, men (and women) consistently rate images with makeup as more attractive, confident, feminine and healthy.

Makeup doesn't merely change how men view a woman's looks. When asked to evaluate personalities, men also give higher scores to women who wear makeup. Furthermore, waitresses wearing makeup earn higher tips from their male clientèle. Studies show that men think women who wear makeup have higher-status jobs and are more intelligent, confident, interesting and efficient!

Dr. Nicolas Guéguen, from Université de Bretagne-Sud, even asserts that women who wear makeup in bars are more likely to receive attention from males. He found that men approached a woman sooner and more often when she wore makeup than when she didn't. However, Guéguen surmises that makeup's effect may not be just because it makes faces look 'prettier'. 'Perhaps the effect of makeup is not to enhance physical attractiveness per se,' he wrote, 'but to serve as a cue to males that 'this female might be available.'

Whatever it is that gives makeup such power, it works – and not only on men. Women feel prettier when they're wearing makeup. A study of American college students found that women had higher opinions of their own bodies and appearance when made up. Putting on cosmetics has been shown to boost self-image in a variety of different women, from the elderly to surgery patients.

It is no wonder that people spend literally billions of dollars annually on makeup. Women are attracted to makeup because it draws upon their innate drive to enhance their femininity, set them apart from men and demonstrate that they are a desirable partner—whether or not they are conscious that this is their motivation.

Alternatives to makeup

Technology continues to advance rapidly. These days, cosmetic procedures can address issues pertaining to the human face. Peels, scrubs and laser treatments can even out skin tone, remove blemishes, rearrange facial fat and tighten skin. Cosmetic tattoos offer replenished color and contrast. Surgery and dermal fillers can correct asymmetry, and so on.

This book, and its sequel, discusses these alternatives.

ATTRACTIVENESS VS BEAUTY

Beauty does not automatically mean attractiveness. We are attracted to people for a wide range of reasons that go beyond their skin texture or bone structure. Attractiveness is more than just finding someone physically appealing.

If it's evolution that drives us, why can't we all simply agree on who is beautiful and who is not? When you talk about individuals, it gets a little more complicated. Evolution explains why we find certain attributes attractive—to a degree. Factors like voice, facial expression, body language, personality and even scent also enhance one's appeal, meaning physical features only take you so far before your inner beauty shines through.

Physical attraction may play a significant role when we first meet someone, but there is more to attraction than meets the eye. Simply being friendly and nice plays an important part in attraction. People who aren't stereotypically good-looking appear attractive to those who know and like them. Researchers asked subjects to evaluate each other before and after working together in groups. In general, likeable people were described as more beautiful because of their happy persona.

Beyond kindness, other traits that make people attractive are cooperativeness and a sense of humor. Being friendly and out-going and making an effort to get along with others all go a long way towards making you seem more attractive to others whilst also boosting the quality of your relationships.

People who can communicate in an expressive and animated way tend to be more liked compared with those who are difficult-to-read. This is because we are more confident in our reading of them and they are therefore less of a threat.

Research shows that two people who share similar interests, values, likes and dislikes feel drawn to each other. People can also feel attracted to others who share a similar physical appearance, background, or personality.

Psychology professor Albert Mehrabian suggests that there are three important elements that account differently for our liking of a person. He calls these as the three Vs – verbal, vocal and visual.[11]

93% of expression is non-verbal. Our actual words make up only 7% of communication, while 38% comes from tone of voice, and 55% comes from our body language. One more element, however, does play a part in our attractiveness to other human beings, and that is smell.

Smell and attractiveness

Certain body odors are connected to human sexual attraction, according to research. Again, this relates back to the innate drive to perpetuate the human race. Subconsciously, by way of scent, humans can discern whether a potential mate will pass on favorable genetic traits to their offspring.

'Research on human mating has found that the effect of scent on males and on females differs. Part of this difference is caused by the different motives each gender holds for mating. Males, in order to pass on genes, subconsciously notice and are attracted to traits that indicate fertility in females, such as a voice of higher pitch, a specific hip-to-waist ratio, and a certain body odor. Evolutionarily, females have two main motives for mating: to pass on genes and to find a partner who can provide adequate support for herself and future offspring. As a female reaches the fertile stage of her menstrual cycle, the desire to pass on

11   *Swami, V., and Furnham, A. (2008). The Psychology of physical attraction. London: Routledge.*

favorable traits to offspring gains more importance and the female becomes more attracted than usual to males with favorable traits. Many such traits are subliminally detected through scent.'[12]

Evolutionary biologist Randy Thornhill of the University of New Mexico found that men with symmetrical facial features even smell better to women. In some cases, women in Thornhill's study reported that they could not smell anything on a man's sweaty shirt, yet they were, nonetheless, attracted to it. 'We think the detection of these types of scent is way outside consciousness,' Thornhill said.

This attraction to scent goes beyond pheremones. Scientific American journalist Adam Hadhazy writes, 'Humans might use a nuanced concoction of chemicals even more complex than formal pheromones to attract potential mates.' [13]

If this is so, then men who wish to be attractive to women might do better to refrain from using 'masculine fragrances' such as after-shave!

Kate Fox in 'The Smell Report' writes: 'Widely publicised research findings on female sensitivity to male pheromones have also led some men to believe that the odor of their natural sweat is highly attractive to women.

'Women are indeed highly sensitive to male pheromones, particularly around ovulation, but many popular assumptions about the effects of these pheromones are the result of misinterpretation and over-simplification of the research results.

'All male pheromones are not equally attractive, and some of the myths stem from an understandable confusion over their names. The male pheromone *androstenone* is not the same as *androstenol*. Androstenol is the scent produced by fresh male sweat, and is attractive to females. Androstenone is produced by male sweat after exposure to oxygen – i.e. when less fresh – and is perceived as highly unpleasant by

---

12   'Body odor and subconscious human sexual attraction.' Wikipedia. Retrieved 28th October 2014
13   'Do Pheromones Play a Role in Our Sex Lives?' By Adam Hadhazy. Scientific American. February 13, 2012.

females (except during ovulation, when their responses change from 'negative' to 'neutral').

'So, men who believe that their 'macho', sweaty body-odor is attractive to women are deluding themselves, unless they are constantly producing fresh sweat and either naked or changing their clothes every 20 minutes to remove any trace of the oxidized sweat.'

Everyone has a different opinion as to what smells are pleasing. Some tribes prefer the smell of cows, or the smell of onions, to any other.[14] The sense of smell is powerful and primitive. Smells can evoke vivid images and emotions and even influence people's moods. Unconsciously, we can even be attracted to the smell of people with the same political beliefs![15]

The part of the human brain that interprets smell is in the brain's limbic system, an area so intimately entwined with memory and feeling that it is sometimes referred to as the 'emotional brain'.

In spite of this biological wiring, however, smells would not awaken memories and emotions if we did not accumulate learned responses. The first time you smell a new scent, you (consciously or unconsciously) associate it with an experience, a person, an object or even an instant in time. Your brain creates a link between the smell and a memory; for example associating the smell of lavender with your grandmother, or a certain aftershave with a school principal you disliked, or the smell of sunscreen with the beach. When you experience the smell again, the connection awakens that particular memory or mood. Lavender might call up a specific grandmother-related memory or simply make you feel content. A whiff of aftershave might make you feel anxious or angry without your understanding the reason. This partly explains why people have different preferences in smells. One female acquaintance of

---

14   Fox, Kate. "The Smell Report." Social Issues Research Centre. (Sept. 20, 2010). http://www.sirc.org/publik/smell.pdf

15   Assortative Mating on Ideology Could Operate Through Olfactory Cues. Rose McDermott, Dustin Tingley and Peter K. Hatemi. American Journal of Political Science, Volume 58, Issue 4, pages 997–1005, October 2014. DOI: 10.1111/ajps.12133 ©2014, Midwest Political Science Association

mine finds herself attracted to men who smell of machine oil, because during her teens she happily dated a youth whose hobby was tinkering with his motorcycle!

Because it is during our youth that we experience most new smells, odors frequently awaken childhood memories. The fact is, however, that we actually start to link smells and emotion even before we are born! Infants who were exposed to certain smells when they were still embryos in the womb, show a liking for the smells.[16]

It is difficult to know what memories, emotions or cultural responses certain external smells can call up in other people. One thing is for certain however: our own personal–clean and hygienic–natural odor, whether or not we are conscious of its existence, is going to be attractive to numerous people, and not infrequently. So avoid the strong perfumes—you may be masking your own subtle, attractive, natural scent!

In conclusion - we can change our appearance with makeup and cosmetic procedures, with manipulation of our body and scalp hair; with clothing, tattoos and adornments; but appearance is only part of the story. Of all the elements that make us attractive to others, beauty is only one.

16   'Long-term flavor recognition in humans with prenatal garlic experience'. Peter G. Hepper1, Deborah L. Wells, James C. Dornan and Catherine Lynch. DOI: 10.1002/dev.21059 Copyright © 2012 Wiley Periodicals, Inc. Developmental Psychobiology, Volume 55, Issue 5, pages 568–574, July 2013

Part 1:
Face Issues

FACE ISSUES: SIGNS OF AGING

Below is a list of the common signs of aging. Please refer to our face therapies section on page 105 to find appropriate treatments.

Deep wrinkles

Deep grooves and wrinkles can be treated with laser, dermal fillers, plasma laser or injections of platelets. Learn more in the section on 'Face Therapy,' page 105.

Discolored teeth

Tooth enamel wears away over time, exposing darker colors and stains of yellow and brown. Pharmacies and drugstores sell brush-on whitening gels. There are also professional teeth whitening treatments available. Learn more by reading the companion book in this series, *Ultimate Beauty 2: Hair, Body and Smile*.

Drooping brows

Drooping eyebrows and wrinkled, sagging forehead skin can make people appear older, tired, sad or angry. These issues can be corrected with surgical 'brow lifts' or with non-invasive methods. See our section on drooping brows, page 26.

Drooping jowls

As we age the fat pads in our cheeks may drop below our jawline, making the face look 'square'. See our section on jawline and neck rejuvenation under 'Face Therapy' (page 165).

Dry skin

As we age, our skin generally becomes drier. See our section on dry skin under 'Skin Issues' (page 41).

Fine lines and wrinkles

A loss of collagen and elastin reduces skin volume, causing fine lines and wrinkles. Repeated muscle motions—laughing, squinting, eating and drinking—etch crow's-feet around the eyes and marionette lines near the mouth.

Prevention is the best treatment. Always wear a sunscreen when outdoors. Practice a regular skin car routine, incorporating antioxidants and retinoids. See our section on Basic Skin Care (page 187).

A medical practitioner can provide treatments like wrinkle-relaxing injections, dermal fillers, and laser therapy. Usually wrinkle-relaxers such as Botox are used for the upper part of the face (forehead lines, that crinkle between your eyes) and dermal fillers are used for the lower half (laugh lines, thin lips).

Long, drooping nose

As we get older our noses tend to droop, because soft tissue (skin, fat, and muscle) relaxes and structural support changes. Bone recedes over time, so there's less foundation to support the skin and cartilage. Furthermore, loss of elasticity and collagen in the skin causes sagging. You cannot really prevent your nose from drooping, but you can minimize the effect by avoid the sun, smoking, and weight fluctuation. Use prescription-strength skincare products, including retinoids, which help preserve and regenerate collagen. A surgical 'nose job' (rhinoplasty) can re-shape the nose.

Thinning eyebrows and lashes

Changing hormones thin out the hairs of our eyebrows and lashes. Years of over-tweezing may also damage the eyebrow follicles, making it harder for hairs to grow back. Topical ointments, hair transplants and cosmetic tattooing are some of the possible solutions.

Thinning skin

A loss of collagen leads to a decrease in skin volume. On the backs of the hands, the veins stand out more. On the face, hollows appear beneath the cheek bones. Dermal fillers can plump up hands and faces that have lost collagen. Lasers can stimulate collagen regeneration.

Thin, pale lips
Lack of fullness in lips can be addressed by treatment with inject-able dermal fillers. Color can be restored with cosmetic tattooing.

'Turkey' neck
Loose, wobbling skin hanging from the neck makes us look older, Fraxel laser treatments can improve the skin's texture, while wrinkle relaxing injections such as Botox can soften vertical lines. Some doctors use Thermage®, ReFirme®, radiofrequency or Intense Pulsed Light devices, to stimulate production of collagen in the neck.

Uneven skin tone
The treatment of skin discoloration, pigmentation and vitiligo issues requires initial assessment and diagnosis by a doctor. Therapies include treatment with laser and/or topical skin products (such as creams). See our section on skin discoloration under 'Skin Issues', page 41.

FACE ISSUES: DROOPING BROWS AND EYELIDS

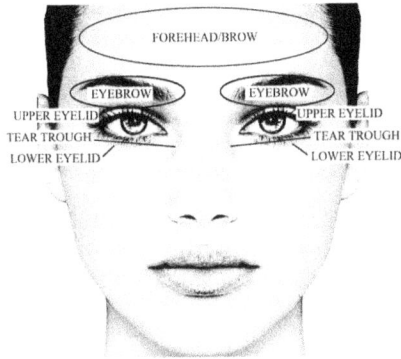

Stress, sun exposure, aging and gravity all contribute to loss of skin elasticity, causing wrinkles and lines in the brow (forehead). Combined with drooping eyebrows, these forehead creases can make people appear older than they actually are, or tired, depressed or angry.

The older we get, the more likely it is that the tissue between the eyebrows and the upper eyelids will also begin to sag, particularly at the outer edges.

The lower lids may appear baggy or puffy, and the hollows beneath them may deepen. As we age, the amount of fat in our lower eyelids actually increases. The tissues and some of the muscles around the eyes weaken, allowing the normal fat inside the eyelids to droop.

Baggy lower eyelids are accentuated by the 'tear trough'. Tear troughs are the hollows beneath the eyes; the grooves running along the junction between the lower eyelid and the cheek. The troughs usually deepen and widen as years go by, creating shadows that make the face look weary.

The eyebrows themselves also change; the hairs may lose color, lengthen and/or become sparser.

SURGERY TO REJUVENATE THE FOREHEAD

Cosmetic surgery techniques (browplasty) can lift drooping brows. Early methods used to involve the surgeon cutting along the hairline, then pulling the skin of the forehead up and back to raise the brows.

These days, brow lifting is often performed by way of keyhole surgery. This is called an 'endoscopic brow lift'. Endoscopic brow lifts may also be fixed in place with a bioabsorbable implant known as an 'Endotine'.

Brow or upper eyelid surgery can also be performed using a laser to cut through the skin. The risk of bleeding is thus decreased.

A number of surgical approaches are used for lifting the forehead. These are discussed in more detail in the section on brow lifting, under 'Face Therapy', page 112.

SURGERY TO REJUVENATE EYELIDS

'Blepharoplasty' is the term used to describe the surgical rejuvenation of the upper or lower eyelids, or both. This procedure usually involves the surgical removal of fat and excess tissue from the eyelids.

A minimally-surgical technique to improve the look of 'hooded' upper eyelids is called the 'Ten Minute Eyelift'. It involves the surgeon running a heated cautery probe along the 'hooded' area of each lid. The skin contracts in response to the heat and the drooping portion draws back.

MINIMALLY INVASIVE TREATMENTS TO REJUVENATE BROWS AND EYELIDS

A non-surgical eyebrow lift can be achieved, although the results are not as dramatic as the results of surgery. Techniques include:

- *Wrinkle relaxing injections.* Careful positioning of anti-wrinkle injections (e.g. Botox or Dysport) into the orbicularis oculi (the muscle around the eyes) provides a lifting effect to the eyebrows by releasing them from the muscle's downward tugging. The improvement is only small, but it can make a noticeable and pleasing difference.

- *Dermal fillers.* A dermal filler injected beneath the eyebrow gives support to the brow and pushes it up. The filler also helps to soften the bony orbital rim around the eyebrows, giving a softer, rejuvenated look. Dermal fillers can also be injected into the middle section of the upper lid/brow to help lift sagging eyelids.

MINIMALLY INVASIVE TREATMENTS TO REJUVENATE LOWER EYELIDS AND TEAR TROUGHS.

Injectable dermal fillers are often used to fill out under-eye troughs. This treatment must be carried out by a qualified doctor, to avoid possible nerve damage in this sensitive area of the face. Some practitioners prefer to avoid this method because of the risk of creating 'bags' of filler in the tender tissues beneath the eye.

PHP (Platelet Rich Plasma) injections may be used to improve the appearance of lower eyelids and tear troughs. Sometimes a combination of techniques is used, such as PRP injections, followed by microneedling, followed by infusion with hyaluronic acid.

NON-SURGICAL TREATMENTS TO REJUVENATE BROWS AND EYELIDS

- *Laser skin therapies:* Laser treatments, such as skin peels, can minimize the appearance of wrinkles in the forehead and tighten the skin a little, but the results are very subtle.
- *PRP injections:* Platelet Rich Plasma injections are recommended for people whose brow area is not drooping or sagging severely. The growth factors in platelets help rejuvenate and regenerate tissue and bone, so that the brow becomes fuller and its appearance is improved.

FACE ISSUES: EYEBROWS

Many estheticians consider the eyebrows to be the most important facial feature. They do play a major role in framing the eyes and they can influence the perceived shape of the face. The shape, color, thickness and position of eyebrows can affect the appearance of facial symmetry, width, and youthfulness; eyebrows can make the eyes appear wider, shapelier or smaller; they can make your expression seem angry, surprised or happy.

Eyebrow shape

When considering how best to groom your eyebrows, it is best not to follow passing trends. As the over-plucked, shaved and high-arched eyebrow shapes of the past have demonstrated, eyebrow styles go in and out of fashion. Instead, tailor your eyebrows to suit your face.

In general, square-shaped faces suit thicker, stronger eyebrows; heart-shaped faces are flattered by 'rounded' eyebrows; flattish/horizontal brows seem to add width to a long face; arched brows are said to make round faces look less round, and almost any style will suit an oval face.

- *Distance between:* Typically, the distance between the eyebrows should equal the width of the nostrils, so ideally you would remove any stray hairs growing in this space between the eyebrows.
- *End points:* To mark the end points of your eyebrows, lay a ruler or other straight object on an angle against your cheek so that one point touches the bottom of your nose and another point reaches the outer corner of your eye. The spot where the ruler intersects your eyebrow is where the hairs, preferably, should end.
- *Thickness:* The ideal eyebrows are between 6 mm (¼ inch) and 12 mm (½ inch) at their thickest. Beginning just below the fullest part of your eyebrow, use an eyeliner pencil to draw a line along the bottom edge of your eyebrow. The line should run above any stray out-of-place hairs, and should follow the natural path of your brow's top edge. This may be

angled, slightly curved, or even straight. Remove the stray hairs from below the line. After the peak of the eyebrow's arch, the eyebrow's tail should be a little slimmer than the main part of the brow, tapering off at the end.

- *Arch*: When you look at yourself straight on, in a mirror, the perfect eyebrow arch should reach its highest point above the outer rim of your iris and lie precisely along your brow bone.

Eyebrow issues can include
- asymmetry of shape and/or position
- unsuitable shape
- thinning of hair
- wiry hairs
- fading color
- gaps or scars
- hairs too long
- awkward positioning
- lack of definition

EYEBROW ENHANCEMENTS

The following treatments do not lift the forehead; however they can improve the appearance of the eyebrows.
- cosmetic tattooing
- snipping/trimming with scissors
- eyebrow transplant
- plucking, shaving
- threading
- waxing
- electrolysis
- eyebrow tinting

Learn more by visiting the section on eyebrow treatments, under 'Face Therapy', page 105.

FACE ISSUES: FACE SHAPE

The shape of your face changes as you age. Changes include drooping jowls, saggy brows, baggy eyes, drooping nose, hollow cheeks, wrinkles, creases and an ill-defined jawline. A once heart-shaped or diamond-shaped face may take on a square or rectangular appearance. A round face may look long.

The most dramatic rejuvenation of face shape is brought about by cosmetic surgery - the 'facelift' and the 'nose job'. Facelifts and nose jobs can be performed in several ways—to learn more, visit the section on facelift surgery on page 130. Fat transfer can also be performed to alter face shape.

Minimally invasive and non-surgical techniques to restore a youthful face shape include injectable dermal fillers, injectable wrinkle relaxants, liposuction, ultrasound and laser therapy, and thread lifting. Learn more by visiting the section 'Face Therapy', page 105.

CONTOURING MAKEUP

HEART-SHAPED   LONG   SQUARE

ROUND   DIAMOND   OVAL

To help you balance or alter the appearance of your face shape, you can use a number of contouring and highlighting tricks with makeup. Products used to achieve this 'sculpted and defined' effect include foundation, blush, bronzers and highlighters. The idea is to paint the bridge of the nose, the tops of the cheekbones, the 'cupid's bow' of the lips, the center of the forehead and the chin, a strip of skin just beneath the eyebrows and any shadowy creases with a light-colored foundation, bronzer or highlighter to make them appear to project forward. A slightly darker shade of foundation is used to paint 'shadows' on the undersides of the cheekbones, the eyelid creases, the sides of the nose and the jawline, to make them appear to recede, giving a 'slimming' effect.

FACE ISSUES: JAWLINE AND NECK

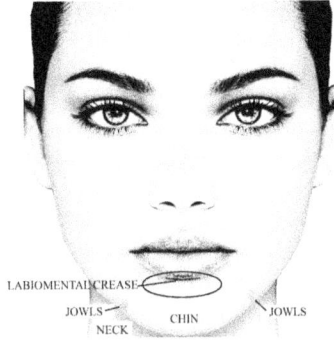

LABIOMENTAL CREASE
JOWLS   JOWLS
CHIN
NECK

JAWLINE AND JOWLS

As we grow older poor facial muscle tone, loss of skin elasticity and facial volume, saggy skin, weight loss or weight gain, genes, sleeping positions, repetitive mouth movements and bad habits such as smoking can lead to the appearance of 'jowls'. Our facial fat pads droop, the face loses roundness and we can end up with areas of facial skin or facial fat that have descended to hang along or below the jaw line. A once-triangular face has now turned into a square face. Soft, irregular flesh replaces a firm, youthful jawline.

When the clean, straight jawline disappears the new, jowly face generally makes people look older. Until recently the only ways we could fight the effects of time on our faces involved surgical facelifts, with results that often resulted in an unnatural, 'stretched' appearance. These days there are many more options.

NECK AND DÉCOLLETAGE

The neck is also an important area to rejuvenate, because your age is often judged by the appearance of your neck. The neck is subject to a number of degenerative changes such as loss of collagen and elastin and accumulation of fat. External factors such as wind, pollution and ultraviolet radiation play a major part.

The neck and the décolletage area are particularly prone to premature aging because these are areas of increased sun exposure.

Traditionally, neck rejuvenation has been performed surgically to help to reposition lax skin, decrease wrinkles and reduce redundant fatty tissues.

Non-surgical procedures can also address the skin texture of the neck and décolletage, whereas surgical procedures are unable to address this issue. Non-surgical jawline and neck rejuvenation can involve minimally invasive procedures with little or no downtime.

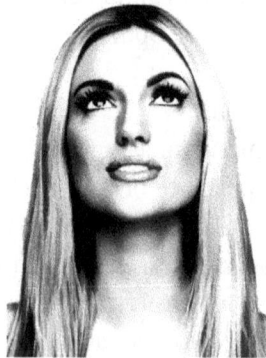

FACE ISSUES: WRINKLES AND LINES

THE LANGUAGE OF WRINKLES

Forehead wrinkles

Frown lines
between brows

Droopy eyebrows

Vertical lip lines

Thin lips

Sagging mouth corners

Undefined jawline

Turkey neck

Crow's feet (periorbital lines)

Sunken trear troughs
beneath eyes

Bunny lines

Deep nasolabial folds

Hollow cheeks

Marionette lines
(Oral commissures)

Sagging jowls

Mental crease

Wrinkles and lines (and sagging skin) are caused by reduced skin elasticity due to such factors as aging, sun exposure, repetitive facial expressions, habitually sleeping on your face, lifestyle and pollution. Wrinkles, lines and loss of elasticity can be addressed with the use of injectable dermal fillers and muscle/wrinkle relaxers, light therapies, chemical peels and topical treatments.

SURGICAL WRINKLE TREATMENTS
Fat Transfer

Your own body fat can be harvested from one area of the body and transferred to another.

Skin Needling

The technique involves rolling a skin needling device over the treatment area. Tiny needles puncture the skin multiple times. This treatment triggers the production of new collagen in the skin. Read more about it on page 238.

MINIMALLY INVASIVE WRINKLE TREATMENTS
Dermal Fillers

Dermal fillers can be injected into the skin to plump it up, increase volume and minimize the appearance of lines and wrinkles. Learn more on page 162.

Wrinkle Relaxers (Botulinum Toxin Type A)

An injection of Botox or Dysport, which are purified versions of the Botulinum toxin A, relaxes the muscle just underneath the wrinkle, allowing the skin on top to lie smooth and crease-free. See page 183.

Laser Resurfacing

Here, energy from a light source—either a laser or a pulsed diode light—removes the top layer of skin, causing a slight but unnoticeable skin "wounding." This kicks the skin's natural collagen-production system into high gear, resulting in smoother, more wrinkle-free skin. See page 206 for more information.

Chemical Peels

In this treatment, one of a variety of different chemicals is used to 'burn' away the top layer of skin, creating damage that causes the body to respond by making more collagen. You end up with younger-looking, smoother skin. Learn more on page 194.

Dermabrasion and Microdermabrasion

A vacuum suction device used in tandem with a mild chemical crystal, dermabrasion helps remove the top layer of skin cells and bring new, more evenly textured skin to the surface. In the process, fine lines and wrinkles seem to disappear. Find out more on page 202.

Plasma Skin Regeneration

Plasma skin regeneration (PSR), is a non-laser treatment that uses a device to deliver energy in the form of a gas called 'plasma' to rejuvenate and tighten skin, improving facial lines and wrinkles and skin pigmentation associated with sun damage. See page 225 for more.

PRP Injections

PRP contains and releases a number of different growth factors and other natural healing cells in your own blood that encourage the healing and regeneration of skin and bone. See page page 228.

Skin Tightening Injections
To tighten the skin and counteract the aging process, poly-L lactic acid is injected into the deep layer of the skin. See page 242 for more.

NON-SURGICAL WRINKLE TREATMENTS
Radiofrequency, radiowave, photodynamic therapy, ultrasound, vacuum suction, IPL (intense pulsed light) and ultraviolet skin therapies can be used to treat wrinkles. Learn more by visiting the relevant topics under 'Face Therapy'. Topical treatments are also useful.

Topical Wrinkle Treatments
Collagen.
Many skin care products are touted as containing collagen. Unfortunately, collagen molecules are too large to be absorbed into the skin, so collagen creams are not very efficacious. Taking collagen orally is not helpful either, because very little collagen can be absorbed by the digestive system. A better approach is to apply ingredients that can encourage new collagen production in the skin, such as vitamin C.

Clinical studies reveal that the following ingredients can reduce wrinkles and lines. Most are found in a variety of skin-care treatments, both prescription and over-the-counter.[17]

Alpha-hydroxy acids (AHAs)
These natural fruit acids lift away the top layer of dead skin cells, reducing the appearance of wrinkles and lines, particularly around the eyes. New evidence shows that in higher concentrations, AHAs may help stimulate collagen production. Natural alpha hydroxy acids include lactic acid (found in milk), glycolic acid (sugar cane), malic acid (apples and pears), citric acid (oranges and lemons) and tartaric acid (grapes). In addition to reducing the appearance of wrinkles, regular use of AHAs can work to even out mottled skin tone and fade age spots.

HOME-MADE AHA FACIAL MASK

17   Source: WebMD.com. Information retrieved December 2014

Can't afford expensive creams? Make your own facial masks. Visit our 'Recipes' section on page 250.

Retinoids (including Retin A).

The only FDA-approved[18] topical treatment for wrinkles is tretinoin, known commercially as Retin A. The regular application of prescription creams containing this ingredient can reduce wrinkles and lines, and repair sun damage.

Retinol is a natural form of vitamin A found in many over-the-counter products. Studies show that in a stabilized formula, in high concentrations, it may be as effective as Retin A, without the side effects such as skin burning and sensitivity.

HOME-MADE RETINOL SERUM
Make your own retinol serum at home. Visit our 'Recipes' section on page 250.

Topical Vitamin C

Studies at Tulane University, among others, have found that vitamin C can increase collagen production, protect against damage from UVA and UVB rays, correct pigmentation problems, and ameliorate inflammatory skin conditions. The type of vitamin C used is very important. Most of the research indicates that the L-ascorbic acid form is the most potent for wrinkle relief.

HOME-MADE VITAMIN C SERUM
Make your own vitamin C serum at home. Visit our 'Recipes' section on page 250.

Idebenone.

---

18   *The FDA is the U. S. Food and Drug Administration. It is responsible for protecting and promoting public health in the U.S.A. through the regulation and supervision of prescription and over-the-counter pharmaceutical drugs (medications), biopharmaceuticals, cosmetics and more.*

This chemical cousin to the nutrient coenzyme Q10 (CoQ10) is a super-powerful antioxidant. In one study published in the Journal of Dermatology, doctors found that with just 6 weeks of topical use there was a 26% reduction in skin roughness and dryness, a 37% increase in hydration, a 29% decrease in lines and wrinkles, and a 33% overall improvement in sun-damaged skin. Other studies have found similar results.

Growth Factors.
Part of the body's natural wound-healing response, these compounds, when applied topically to the skin, may reduce sun damage and decrease lines and wrinkles, while stimulating collagen production.

Pentapeptides.
The results of a study supported by the National Institutes of Health suggested pentapeptides can increase collagen production in sun-damaged skin. Several subsequent studies (including one presented at a national dermatology conference) affirmed that when topically applied, pentapeptides stimulated the skin's collagen production and diminished lines and wrinkles.[19]

Anti-aging skin serums tailored to your DNA
A range of skincare products based on a person's individual DNA is being developed by Professor Chris Toumazou at Imperial College, London, UK. Topical application of the product, named 'Geneu', is said to reduce fine lines and wrinkles by up to 30 per cent within 12 weeks.

First, doctors take a cheek swab from the person to be treated, Next, they inject the DNA strands into a handheld microchip device, which sequences the DNA within 30 minutes. The results are used to tailor the serum to suit the individual. The serum is administered over a four-week period. Its ingredients include white mulberry root extract, vitamins A and C, red baron grass, tripeptides, and collagen-boosting amino acids.

TIPS TO STAVE OFF WRINKLES AND LINES

19   Ibid.

To keep your skin smooth and minimize wrinkles and lines,

- Regularly apply moisturizer.
- Wear a good sun screen.
- Avoid sun exposure between 10am and 3pm.
- Wear sunglasses to preserve the delicate skin around the eyes.
- Do not smoke.
- Avoid pollution.
- Eat fresh fruits and vegetables.
- Cultivate good sleeping habits.
- Don't squint too often.
- Do not sleep with your face pressed into the pillow.

FACE ISSUES: EYELASHES

Eyelashes can enhance the look of the eyes and the face. Problems with the appearance of eyelashes can include:

- lack of eyelashes
- sparse lashes
- over-short lashes
- over-long lashes
- lashes that are an unwanted color

These issues can generally be addressed with treatments such as prosthetics, makeup, cosmetic tattooing and prescription drugs. See our sections on eyebrow and eyelash treatments under 'Face Therapy,' page 105.

Trichotillomania, also known as trichotillosis or hair pulling disorder, is condition characterized by the compulsive urge to pull out one's hair. This may include the eyelashes. Trichotillomania can lead to psychological distress, and the impairment of one's social life. Treatments include medications and psychotherapy.

Part 2:
Skin Issues

SKIN ISSUES: HUMAN SKIN

The skin is the largest organ of the body, with a total area of about 1.8 square metres (20 square feet). Our skin safeguards us from bacteria and other microorganisms, protects us from the elements, helps regulate body temperature, and allows the sensations of touch, heat, and cold.

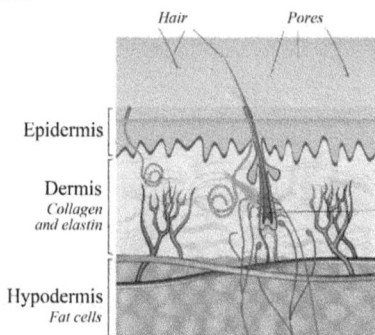

THE SKIN'S THREE LAYERS:

The epidermis
The outermost layer of skin, the epidermis furnishes a waterproof barrier and is responsible for our skin tone. It also houses cells called melanocytes, which produce the pigment 'melanin'. Melanin determines the color of our skin.

The dermis
This layer lies beneath the epidermis. It comprises tough connective tissue, hair follicles and sweat glands. The dermis is a fibrous network of tissue that gives structure and resilience to the skin. On average it is about 0.08 inches (2 mm) thick.

The mesh-like web of the dermis is made of the structural proteins collagen and elastin, in addition to blood and lymph vessels, mast cells and fibroblasts. These components are enclosed within a gel-like substance called the 'ground substance', composed mostly of molecules called 'glycosaminoglycans'. The ground substance is essential to the skin's hydration and moisture levels. Both collagen and elastin are manufactured in cells called fibroblasts, most of which exist in the upper surface of the dermis where it joins the epidermis.

The hypodermis
This deeper tissue beneath the dermis is composed of fat and connective tissue.

COLLAGEN AND ELASTIN

Collagen and elastin are two biological substances that occur naturally in our skin. Together they are responsible for the skin's strength, firmness, and shape. The process of aging depletes the skin of these two important proteins.

Collagen
'Collagen' is the term for a group of proteins that mostly occur in the connective or 'fibrous' tissues of the dermis. They are the most common proteins in the human body, comprising around 30 percent of total protein content. Collagen is abundant in our skin, but is also part of our ligaments, blood vessels, bones, and eyes.

Connective tissues support and/or connect various forms of tissues or body organs. Their role is to strengthen other tissues and support their shape. Some examples of connective tissues include cartilage, fat and tendons.

Elastin
Like collagen, elastin is also a protein located in connective tissues. It is, however, a different type of protein. Elastin is elastic; that is, it enables the body's tissues to 'snap back' to their original shape after they have been contracted or stretched. Elastin can be compared to a rubber band.

Our artery walls, lungs, intestines and skin all contain elastin. All these tissues need to be able to expand and contract to keep us healthy. When young skin containing abundant elastin is pinched or pulled, it resumes its normal shape when released. Elastin is responsible for this. An example of skin stretching occurs when we smile, or make any other facial expression.

It could be said that collagen is for skin structure while elastin is for skin 'bounce'.

These two proteins are important in skin care because their actions combine to give skin its shape and firmness. Collagen provides density, compactness and volume. It is the basic supporting structure, while elastin permits stretched skin to return to the shape collagen gives it.

Collagen is composed of very strong fibers with exceptional tensile strength. These fibers provide the foundation to anchor the skin's outer layer. Elastin is not as abundant in the skin as collagen, but is essential for skin function. It forms an elastic network between the collagen fibers.

When skin is deficient in collagen and elastin it sags and wrinkles. In young skin, collagen and elastin are abundant. Skin looks smooth and taut. During the aging process, the body's production of collagen and elastin decreases. Sun damage, pollution and other factors also contribute to the breaking down of the skin's connective fibers. The skin becomes thinner and even more vulnerable to sun-damage and other environmental aggravations.

The elastin in aging skin begins to lose its ability to snap back, just as a rubber band that is continually stretched will, over time, lose its resilience. When this happens, our skin sags. Usually we notice this most around the eyes, jaw line, and neck.

PROTECTING YOUR SKIN'S COLLAGEN AND ELASTIN

The good news is that you can slow down the skin's aging process.
Here's how:
- Protect your skin's structure and elasticity by using a high
  strength sunscreen daily.
- Regularly apply proven skin care products that nourish it and
  provide antioxidant protection—such as vitamin A and vitamin
  C serum—to minimize the damage caused by free radicals.
- Sloughing off dead skin cells can encourage skin to regenerate.
  Gently exfoliate your skin 2 – 3 times per week.
- Protect your skin with moisturizers.

SIGNS OF AGING SKIN
Below is a list of the common signs of skin aging. Please refer to
our therapies sections to find appropriate treatments—"Face Therapy"
on page 105 and "Skin Therapy" on page 184.

Deep wrinkles

Deep grooves and wrinkles can be treated with laser, dermal fillers,
plasma laser or injections of platelets.

Dry skin

As we age, our skin generally becomes drier. See our section
"Skin Issues: dry skin" on page 66.

Fine lines and wrinkles

A decrease in collagen and elastin reduces skin volume and elasticity, causing fine lines and wrinkles. Repeated muscle motions such
as laughing, squinting, eating and drinking etch crow's-feet around
the eyes and marionette lines near the mouth. Prevention is the best
treatment. Always wear a sunscreen when outdoors. Practice a regular
skin care routine, incorporating antioxidants and retinoids. See our
section on Basic Skin Care, page 187.

Thinning skin

The decrease in skin volume caused by a loss of collagen affects namy parts of the body. On the backs of the hands, the veins stand out more. On the face, hollows appear beneath the cheek bones. Dermal fillers can plump up hands and faces that have lost collagen. Laser therapy can stimulate collagen regeneration.

Uneven skin tone

The treatment of skin discoloration, pigmentation and vitiligo issues requires initial assessment and diagnosis by a doctor. Therapies include treatment with laser and/or topical skin products (such as creams and ointments). See our section on skin pigmentation on page 59.

TREATMENTS FOR SKIN ISSUES

Cosmetic skin therapy offers hope for treating skin issues such as wrinkles, acne and acne scars, skin lesions, blackheads, eczema, enlarged pores, scars, stretch marks and pock marks, sagging skin, varicose veins, spider veins, unsightly tattoos, skin pigmentation, aging skin, psoriasis, vitiligo and more.

Learn more in the section on "Skin Therapy", page 184.

SKIN ISSUES: ACNE AND ACNE SCARRING

ACNE

Acne occurs when the oil-secreting glands in the skin are clogged and become inflamed or infected. This can be caused by or exacerbated by –

- hormones
- stress
- birth control pills
- not enough rest

Symptoms of acne include whiteheads (closed, plugged oil glands), blackheads (open, plugged oil glands), pustules and cysts (large fluid-filled bumps).

The first step in resolving this issue is to clear acne lesions, reduce inflammation and encourage the healing process. This initial stage may take 4–6 weeks depending on the type and frequency of treatments required. Home-care topical formulations, oral vitamin supplements and monthly maintenance treatments should continue to keep the skin clear.

ACNE SCARRING

Even with the most cautious and painstaking therapy, acne scars may still be left behind after acne lesions have been successfully treated. Discolorations are not really acne scars but post-inflammatory hyperpigmentation, which fades as time goes on.

Acne scars can be addressed with a range of non-surgical techniques, depending on the type of scar. For more serious cases, surgery may be necessary. It is vital that you ask your clinician to assess the type of scarring and plan a program specifically for you.

The following risk factors may lead to acne scarring—

- A genetic tendency to scar
- Large size and depth of the lesion
- Naturally slow healing of the skin
- Smoking
- Drinking alcohol
- Poor nutrition
- Poor hydration
- Excess weight/obesity
- Not enough rest
- Improper wound care
- Being slow to identify infection
- Chronic illness
- Stress on your acne lesion wound
- Exposure to sunlight

In general, acne scars can be classified in two categories:
- Indented or depressed – those caused by a loss of tissue (atrophic).
- Raised or thickened – those caused by an excess of tissue (hypertrophic).

Within these categories, acne scars can be sorted into four types: ice pick, boxcar, rolling (which are indented) and keloid scars (which are raised).

TYPES OF ACNE SCARS
Ice Pick Scars
These are deep, very narrow scars that delve into the dermis. The skin looks as if it has been scored by an ice pick or other sharp instrument. Ice pick scars appear to make a small, deep hole in the skin. Some may resemble large, open pores.

SKIN ISSUES: ACNE AND ACNE SCARRING

Ice pick scars develop after an infection from a cyst or other deep inflamed blemish works its way to the surface. The bacteria destroy skin tissue, resulting in a long column-like scar.

This type of scar can be treated with *punch excision* or *punch grafting*. With *punch excision*, the surgeon cuts into the skin with a special punch tool matched to the size of the acne scar, to remove the scar before closing the wound with stitches. The punch tool is somewhat different from conventional plastic surgery cutting tools. It can actually remove tiny fragments of tissue without stretching or affecting the surrounding skin. In *punch grafting* a skin graft, generally removed from behind the ear, is used to stop up the hole in the skin.

Boxcar Scars

Boxcar scars are round or oval dents with steep vertical sides. Wider than ice picks, boxcar scars give the skin a pitted appearance.

When an inflammatory breakout destroys collagen, tissue is lost. The skin over this area is left without support; it sinks and a depressed area appears. Boxcar scars may be superficial to severe, depending on the amount of tissue lost.

Treatments for boxcar scars include punch excision (see above) or punch elevation (see below), dermal fillers, and laser resurfacing.

Punch elevation is a microsurgical method that can be performed in the surgeon's rooms. Using the punch tool, the surgeon commences pinching the scar tissue base. The action of the punch tool resembles pinching-off the scar tissue in a controlled way, to make sure that the underlying skin is minimally affected. When the scar tissue base is sufficiently punched, the base of the acne scar will be level with the outer walls surrounding the scar, i.e. the scar base is 'elevated'. This 'raising' effect makes the scar appear shallower.

Next, the surgeon puts sutures (stitches) into the scar site. Tiny pieces of the surrounding skin are incorporated into the sutures. The result is that the scar site is overlaid by new skin, which in turn triggers the skin's healing.

Rolling Scars

This type of scarring causes 'rolling' or 'wave-like' undulations across skin that otherwise looks normal.

Rolling scars arise when fibrous bands of tissue develop between the skin and the subcutaneous tissue below. These bands pull on the epidermis, binding it to deeper structures of the skin. It is this pulling of the epidermis from within that creates the rolling appearance of the skin.

Rolling scars are best treated with subcision, which is a relatively simple and low risk surgery procedure that can be performed in a day surgery. It is used to treat indented acne scars and may be combined with other therapies such as laser, skin microneedling (e g. 'dermaroller'), punch grafting of the skin (see above), dermabrasion etc.

Hypertrophic or Keloid Scars

A hypertrophic scar looks like a raised, firm mass of tissue. These kinds of scars frequently grow bigger than the original wound. Hypertrophic scars caused by acne are most often found on the torso, especially in men.

Unlike ice pick or boxcar scars, hypertrophic scars are not caused by a loss of tissue. Instead, they develop because of an overproduction of collagen. Steroid (cortisone) creams, tapes, or injections are used to help shrink and flatten the scar. Interferon injections may also be used to soften scar tissue.

TRADITIONAL ACNE MEDICATIONS

There are several drugs which doctors usually prescribe for acne. These include antibiotics, contraceptives, hormones and isotretinoin (Ro-Accutane). Many health professionals are, however, worried about the potential problems and adverse side effects of some of these treatments.

Antibiotics

The use of antibiotics can lead to the development of antibiotic resistance. In the general human population, bacterial resistance has increased drastically during the last few years. Prolonged and widespread use of antibiotics is known to increase the legions of resistant bacteria.

Hormones, contraceptives and isotretinoin.

There is no doubt that hormones and isotretinoin are effective; however using them carries risks. It is mostly teenagers who suffer from acne. At this stage in their growth, young people are emotionally volatile. They may be adversely affected by hormone-based drugs and isotretinoin. Indeed, acne alone is often associated with depression. The effect of emotion-amplifying drugs may have devastating consequences on the roller-coaster moods of young people, and may even cause serious side effects such as depression. If used by pregnant women, they may cause birth defects in the child.

OTHER ACNE TREATMENT OPTIONS

In recent years, breakthroughs in laser and light therapy and clinical treatments have offered alternative solutions for sufferers of acne and acne scarring. The combined use of these therapies, in conjunction with the application of vitamin A creams or ointments, decreases the skin's sebaceous secretion and inflammation. It also reduces the post-inflammatory hyper-pigmentation which is associated with acne scarring.

A disease such as acne, which springs from a number of causes, requires a number of solutions. Various methods may be used to deal with inflammatory lesions, sterilize the skin, reduce follicle blockages, curb sebum production and create a healthy balance in the skin. Such a multifaceted approach may include one or more of the following:

MINIMALLY INVASIVE ACNE AND SCARRING TREATMENTS

- Chemical peels (page 194).
- Medical microdermabrasion (page 202).
- Skin microneedling (page 238).
- Indented scars may require a course of treatment with fractionated laser or skin needling after acne has cleared.
- Moderate to severe acne scarring usually requires either:
  - A course of 3 to 5 skin needling treatments (page 238), or
  - 1 -2 fractionated laser resurfacing treatments (page 206).

NON-SURGICAL ACNE AND SCARRING TREATMENTS

- Red light LED therapy (page 219).
- Laser/ IPL therapy (page 217).
- Topical application of Vitamin A preparations and/or other skincare products (see also "Home-made Skin Care Recipes" on page 250).
- Specific combinations of vitamins and other oral supplements to help clear acne lesions and encourage skin healing..
- Alkaline scar remodeling—Medical alkaline washes, applied to the skin, cause mild irritation. The skin forms a scab over the irritated area. When the scab falls off, the skin tissue has been softened and the scarred area looks smoother.
- Silicone gel sheeting, worn over the scar for a period of time, can effectively prevent and treat of hypertrophic scar and/or keloid formation.
- Enzyme therapy—Topical enzyme treatments can tighten the skin, which in turn smooths out the appearance of scars.

- Chemical peels (see page 194) can not only improve the appearance of scars, they can also help reduce pigmentation, uneven skin color, fine lines, wrinkles, and coarse or uneven texture.
- Mild acne scarring including pigmented marks may respond to one of the following:
  - A course of IPL photorejuvenation (page 217).
  - Laser treatment (page 206)
  - Red light LED treatment (page 219).

Consult with your clinician to work out a therapy program specifically tailored to treat your type of acne and acne scarring.

SKIN ISSUES: BLACKHEADS AND WHITEHEADS

'A comedo is a clogged hair follicle (pore) in the skin. Keratin (sloughed skin debris) combines with oil to block the follicle. A comedo can be open (blackhead) or closed by skin (whitehead), and occur with or without acne. The word *comedo* comes from Latin, to suggest the worm-like look of a blackhead that has been secreted. The plural of comedo is comedones.'[20]

The dark coloring of blackheads is not caused by dirt trapped in the pores or follicles. Instead it is due to oxidation from exposure to the air.

Blackhead and whitehead removal can be achieved by a variety of methods, ranging from at-home treatments to sophisticated cosmetic therapies.

---

20   Source: *Wikipedia. Retrieved August 2014.*

ABOUT PIMPLES

Acne and pimples are closely related. Pimples are comedones that have become inflamed and which have turned into papules or pustules.

Papules are delineated, firm skin bumps, containing no visible fluid and varying in size from a pinhead to 0.4 inches (1 cm) in diameter. They can be brown, purple, pink or red in color.

Pustules are similar small bumps on the epidermis, but filled with fluid or pus caused by infection. The infection is not chronic, as it is with acne.

ABOUT MILIA AND SEBACEOUS FILAMENTS

Comedones are distinct from *sebaceous filaments*, which are miniscule collections of sebum and dead skin cells around hair follicles, and which usually look like small hair-like strands.

Milia is the term for tiny, hard, white bumps that can appear — usually on the face — on anyone of any age, including babies, teens, and adults. They are neither whiteheads nor pimples. These annoying yet harmless lumps usually resolve themselves, but they may last for weeks, months or even years.

MINIMALLY-INVASIVE   TREATMENTS   FOR   BLACKHEADS AND WHITEHEADS

Microdermabrasion and Skin Vacuuming

Microdermabrasion (page 202) is a good option for the removal of blackheads and whiteheads because it is an excellent method of exfoliation. Combined with gentle skin-vacuuming (page 248) it can remove the top layer of dead skin to prevent clogging.

Chemical Peels

Chemical peels (page 194) provide superficial to medium depth exfoliation for blackheads and whiteheads using products that include glycolic acid and lactic acids (AHAs), salicylic acid (BHA), retinoids (vitamin A), resorcinol , mandelic acid, niacinamide (vitamin B3) and enzymes. The appropriate chemical peel can provide a simultaneous action to decongest, de-clog and disinfect skin affected by blackheads and whiteheads while reducing inflammation and preventing future breakouts.

NON-SURGICAL TREATMENTS FOR BLACKHEADS AND WHITEHEADS

Low Level Laser Therapy (LLLT)
LLLT (page 219) employs a medical grade 'cold laser' to decrease blackhead and whitehead formation and severity without heat or discomfort. A course of LLLT treatments will make the complexion clearer and smoother, reducing pore congestion.

Laser Treatment and Light Treatment
Laser, Intense Pulsed Light, and radiofrequency devices are used to treat blackheads and whiteheads, with and without the use of photodynamic therapy. See "Skin Therapy: laser skin therapies" on page 206, Intense Pulsed Light (IPL) on page 217, "Radiofrequency Skin Tightening" on page 154 and "Skin Therapy: photodynamic therapy" on page 224.

AT-HOME TREATMENTS
A regular skin care routine is the best way to avoid getting blackheads in the first place. It can also help get to rid of them.

- Always remove your make-up and cleanse your skin before bedtime. Avoid squeezing blackheads with your fingers, because it can cause scarring and infection.
- Avoid 'comedogenic' skin care products that congest your pores.
- Some people like to use a konjac sponge to cleanse their skin[21].
- Include fresh fruit and vegetables in your diet and drink plenty of water.

Learn how to make your own cleansers, exfoliating scrubs and other skin care products in our "Recipes" section (page 250).

---

21   *The Japanese konjac sponge is a made from the natural fibers of the vegetable 'konjac' ('konnyaku'). These gentle but effective sponges have been used in Japan for more than a century, to cleanse and exfoliate the skin. Many konjac sponges sold commercially are impregnated with additional compounds such as charcoal, green tea, rose extract and clay.*

Step by step guide to blackhead and whitehead removal at home:

- *Cleanse* – Every night before bed, wash your face to get rid of makeup, oil and grime. Clean the skin using cotton pads or sponges and a gentle cleanser specific to your skin type – i.e. normal, dry, oily, sensitive, etc.

  Note: some people prefer to use an electric face brush to remove dirt from their skin. These beauty tools are brushes with a vibrating heads, used on damp skin in conjunction with a gel cleanser. The manufacturers claim that they clean, refresh, massage and exfoliate the skin, removing more grime than hands or a washcloth, stimulating the circulation, balancing oily and dry patches and even improving the appearance of skin blemishes. When the skin is cleaner, skin-care formulations such as such as moisturizers, serums and masks penetrate more effectively. Studies funded by electric face brush manufacturers support these claims—however, there have been no independent studies. Over-enthusiastic use of an electric face brush can strip the skin of its natural oils and cause inflammation. People with sensitive skin should use such tools with caution.

- *Steam* – cover your face with a steaming hot (not uncomfortably hot), damp face-washer. Leave it on for a few minutes and repeat if desired, until the skin is warm. Taking a hot shower or bath has the same effect. Steaming opens the pores, but it can cause broken capillaries and discoloration if done on sensitive skin, or if the steam is too hot, so be careful.

- *Extract* – use a sterilized stainless steel *comedo extraction tool*, according to the instructions included in the packet. These metal implements with looped ends are available from drugstores and pharmacies. If you do not have access to such a tool, thoroughly wash and sanitize your hands. Clip your fingernails short and blunt and cover them with clean, white tissue paper before gently squeezing the skin to extract impurities. Some people use pore strips to unclog the pores in the nose. Do not use pore strips more often than twice a week at the most.

- *Scrub* – if your skin is not delicate or sensitive, use a 'mechanical' exfoliant. This type of exfoliation can be performed using microfiber cloths, adhesive exfoliation sheets, facial scrubs made with sugar or salt crystals, or gently abrasive materials such as sponges, loofahs or brushes. Facial scrubs are available as over-the-counter products.[22] Be careful not to overdo this scrubbing step or you risk skin damage.

  Important note: Avoid any commercial products containing 'microbeads'. Because they are too small (less than 1 mm) to be filtered out by sewage works, tonnes of microbeads are continually released into the environment. The damage to beaches and marine ecosystems is catastrophic.

  In June 2014 the US state of Illinois became the first to ban the use of microbeads; however companies all over the rest of the world continue to include them as ingredients. As consumers, we can help protect the environment by refusing to buy products containing microbeads, which in any case do not work as well as sugar or salt crystals, since plastic lacks their natural ionic properties.

- *Exfoliate* – using a gentle 'chemical' exfoliating product such as low-concentration salicylic acid, glycolic acid, citric acid, malic acid, alpha hydroxy acids (AHAs), beta hydroxy acids (BHAs), fruit enzymes or an enzymatic peel to remove the dead skin cells clinging to the skin's surface. Do not over-exfoliate, and do not exfoliate more than two to three times per week. We recommend exfoliating after comedone extraction, not

---

22   *Wikipedia, 'Exfoliation (cosmetology)' Article retrieved November 2014.*

before, as exfoliation can make the skin very tender. If you have sensitive skin, test the formulation on a small area of skin first, before applying it to your entire face.

- *Nourish and moisturize* – Apply serums, moisturizers and makeup that are 'noncomedogenic' i.e. that will not clog your pores.

- *Soothe* – apply a calming/anti-inflammatory face mask aimed at your skin type (dry, oily, combination, sensitive, mature etc.). This step is optional.

- *Heal* – apply aloe vera gel to the skin. If you keep the gel in the refrigerator it will feel cool and pleasant.

- *Protect* – Cover your face with a high-protection sunscreen several times a day no matter the season of the year. Exfoliation leave your skin more vulnerable to damaging UV rays, which weaken the collagen, leading to sagging skin and enlarged pores.

Perform your blackhead and whitehead removal in the evening, so that the skin has time to recover overnight.

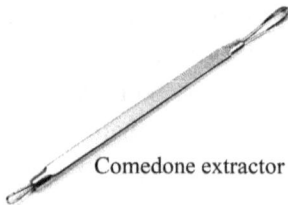

Comedone extractor

SKIN ISSUES: DISCOLORATION OR PIGMENTATION

'Skin pigmentation', also known as 'skin discoloration', is a term used to describe disorders that cause patches of skin to appear lighter or darker than normal, or blotchy and discolored.

Skin discoloration occurs because the body produces either too much or too little melanin, the pigment that gives color to our hair, skin and eyes. Melanin is important to our well-being. It protects the body by absorbing ultraviolet light.

Scientists are still studying the reasons why such skin disorders occur. In some cases there are obvious causes such as sun exposure, drug reactions, hormones, skin trauma or genetic inheritance. In other cases, the reason is not so clear.

Sun Exposure: Pigmentation, appearing as brown patches, can be triggered by ultraviolet (UV) light from the sun. The first method of treating skin pigmentation is to prevent its appearance, or its worsening, by daily application of sunscreen. UV exposure from sunlight or sun beds will invariably worsen any existing pigmentation and promote further pigmentation, so protection from sunlight is essential. The risk of skin cancers also rises with increasing exposure to UV rays.

Dermatologists recommend physical sunscreens as opposed to chemical sunscreens. Physical sunscreens contain titanium dioxide and zinc oxide. These are not absorbed by the skin, and they provide long lasting protection throughout the day.

Chemical sunscreens with chemical ingredients such as para-aminobenzoic acid need reapplication after two hours. They are absorbed into the skin. Studies have found that these chemicals penetrate the bloodstream and can be found in the liver soon after you apply them. There is some debate about whether such products pose a health risk.

Make sure you apply sunscreen liberally, all over the exposed skin, without missing any spots. Sunscreen should be applied every day, even if the day is cloudy, or overcast. As long as there is sunlight to see by, UV light is still present. Avoid direct sunlight, especially during the middle of the day. Seek shade when possible, and wear a hat and protective clothing.

HOME-MADE SUNSCREEN
Make your own sunscreen at home. Visit our 'Recipes' section on page 250.

TYPES OF SKIN DISCOLORATION
Many skin discoloration disorders have specific names. Some examples follow.

Hyperpigmentation

This term refers to the darkening of an area of skin or nails caused by increased melanin.

Vitiligo

Vitiligo is a condition that causes depigmentation of parts of the skin. It occurs when skin pigment cells die or are unable to function. The cause of vitiligo, aside from cases of contact with certain chemicals, is unknown, but research suggests it may arise from autoimmune, genetic, oxidative stress, neural, or viral causes. The incidence worldwide is less than 1%. [23]

Poikiloderma of Civatte

'Poikiloderma of Civatte' is a reddish-brown mottled discoloration on the sides of the neck, which is more commonly seen in women, particularly fair-skinned women.

Poikiloderma is best treated with the Gemini Laser or Pulsed Dye Laser, two of the lasers listed in "Skin Therapy: laser skin therapies" on page 206. This treatment helps to reduce the pigmentation and close off any superficial capillaries causing the redness. The wavelengths from these lasers are specifically attracted to the capillaries and pigmentation, and hence normal skin is relatively unaffected.

23   'Vitiligo'. Wikipedia. Article retrieved November 2014.

Solar (actinic) Keratosis

Solar keratosis lesions are also known as 'actinic' lesions. They look like scaly, red patches on the skin, and they tend to appear after the skin has been regularly exposed to sunlight over a long period, such as several years, because sun damage is cumulative. Fairer skin types are more susceptible to this type of skin discoloration.

The treatment of solar keratosis is more than cosmetic - it is also necessary for good health, because the lesions are pre-cancerous.

Melasma

Melasma is a tan or dark skin discoloration. Although it can affect anyone, melasma is particularly common in women, especially pregnant women (when it is known as 'the mask of pregnancy') and those who are taking contraceptives or hormone replacement therapy (HRT) medications. Melasma is also common in pre-menopausal women. It is thought to be enhanced by surges in certain hormones.

The symptoms of melasma are dark, irregular well-demarcated hyperpigmented spots or patches commonly found on the upper cheek, nose, lips, upper lip, and forehead. These patches often develop gradually over time. Melasma does not cause any other symptoms beyond the discoloration.

Researchers think that melasma is caused by female sex hormones stimulating melanocytes (cells in the epidermal layer of skin that produce the melanin pigment) to produce more melanin pigments when sunlight touches the skin.

Women with a light brown skin type who live in sunny regions are particularly susceptible to developing this condition. It also runs in families and is more common in people with thyroid disease. Stress may be another cause. Other rare causes of melasma include allergic reaction to medications and cosmetics.[24]

---

24   'Melasma'. Wikipedia. Article retrieved November 2014.

Freckles

Freckles are clusters of concentrated melanin which are most often visible on people with a fair complexion. In contrast to lentigines and moles, these spots of color do not have an increased number of melanin producing cells (melanocytes).

Purpura

Flat, purplish patches of skin are called 'purpura'. This condition occurs when tiny blood vessels (capillaries) break, leaking blood into the skin. In older people, the condition is called 'senile purpura' or 'actinic purpura'. Purpura looks like a rash that may appear red at first and gradually turns brown or purple.

There is no specific treatment for this condition. People who have it should avoid vigorous rubbing of the skin, or anything else that may damage the capillaries. Creams that soften the skin may be useful. Some physicians also recommend applying vitamin C serum, but as yet no study has confirmed the efficacy of this.[25]

Lentigines, including sunspots and liver spots.

A lentigo (plural lentigines) is a small pigmented spot on the skin with a clearly defined edge, surrounded by skin that appears normal. It is a harmless increase in the number of melanocytes (skin color cells).

Lentigines are distinct from moles (melanocytic nevi). They are also different from freckles. Freckles have a relatively normal number of melanocytes but an increased amount of melanin. A lentigo has an increased number of melanocytes. Freckles will increase in number and darkness when they receive more sunlight, whereas lentigines will stay the same color regardless of sunlight exposure.[26]

Sunspots or 'solar lentigines' are dark (and sometimes light) patches on the skin. These can be a variety of shapes and colors and develop anywhere on the skin, though they are most common on the

25   'Skin wrinkles and blemishes'. Milton S. Hershey Medical Center. Review Date: 12/18/2012. Reviewed By: Harvey Simon, MD, Editor-in-Chief, In-Depth Reports; Associate Professor of Medicine, Harvard Medical School; Physician, Massachusetts General Hospital. Also reviewed David Zieve, MD, MHA, Isla Ogilvie, PhD, and the A.D.A.M. editorial team.

26   'Lentigo'. Wikipedia. Retrieved November 2014

hands and face. People of all ages are prone to these spots, though lighter skinned individuals are more likely to develop them.

The chief cause of sunspots is constant exposure to sunlight, although yeast, natural pigmentation, fungus and certain skin disorders can also play a part.

Long periods of sun exposure can also increase your risk of damaging your skin and developing skin cancer.

Liver spots are lentigines that are also known as 'sun-induced pigmented lesions'. They look like flat, brown spots on the skin. In spite of their name, they are not associated with the liver. They often appear as we age, and usually on the hands and face. As time passes, liver spots frequently become larger and darker.

Your age, skin type and the amount of time you have spent in the sun without protection will determine how many liver spots appear on your skin, and how big and how dark they become. Liver spots are harmless, but have your skin checked by a doctor every year, because you should beware of *lentigo maligna*, which is an early sign of melanoma. Liver spots are harmless, although most people prefer their skin tone to be even and youthful in appearance. Treatments may include the following:

- Trichloroacetic acid (a chemical peel).
- Tretinoin (retin A) alone, or in combination with mequinol (solage). Tretinoin is a form of vitamin A.
- Professional freezing with liquid nitrogen (cryotherapy).
- Laser treatment is effective in eliminating many liver spots in one treatment. Laser treatment may be more effective than cryotherapy and may have fewer side effects.
- Bleaching creams are widely available, but they are not as effective as a chemical peel. High concentrations of the bleaching ingredient can cause permanent loss of skin color.

TREATMENTS FOR SKIN DISCOLORATION

The treatment of skin discoloration issues requires initial assessment and diagnosis by a doctor.

Discoloration/pigmentation can be treated on any part of the face or body, including the neck, décolletage, back, and back of hands. Therapies include treatment with laser and/or topical skin products such as creams and ointments. The main difference between the two is that lasers can produce a faster and more effective result in most cases. Topical lightening agents usually only fade pigmentation rather than remove it completely.

Different lasers are required for different types of skin pigmentation and skin types. There are however, more risks with the use of lasers as opposed to lightening agents. These risks include worsening of the pigmentation, loss of normal skin pigmentation or scarring of the skin (rare). Also, with laser treatment there is usually a period of recovery post-treatment.

The mode of treatment used will depend on patient preference, patient risk tolerance, and the type of pigmentation treated.

Laser Therapy

Some lasers can be used for the treatment of skin pigmentation and have minimal or no impact on normal skin. This is due to a process called 'selective photothermolysis', in which a particular laser wavelength is mainly attracted to pigmented lesions and hardly attracted at all to the normal skin. This allows selective removal of a lesion. The laser can selectively disrupt the pigment with minimal or no damage to surrounding skin.

One type of laser for treating pigmentation is the millisecond pulse width laser. These lasers emit pulses of light that are attracted to the melanin in the pigment, and this selectively breaks down the pigment by heating it. Examples of this laser include the Gemini Laser and the Candela V-beam pulsed dye laser.

Another type of laser for treating pigmentation is the Q-switched laser. These lasers emit nanosecond pulses (1 nanosecond = 1 billionth of a second) of light that are attracted to the melanin in the pigmented skin. They also selectively heat the pigment to disrupt it, but because the pulses are much shorter, they also have a photomechanical effect— i.e. they shatter and shock the pigment, causing it to break down. It is this effect that allows these lasers to remove tattoo pigment as well.

Generally the advantage of these lasers is that they require fewer sessions to treat pigmentation than the millisecond lasers. It is a more aggressive and effective treatment, and therefore also has more side effects such as a longer recovery time as well as an increased chance of post-inflammatory hyperpigmentation. Examples of these lasers include the Sinon Ruby laser and the Medlite laser.

Learn more about lasers in the section on laser skin therapies under 'Skin Therapy' (page 184).

Cryosurgery/cryotherapy

This method involves using liquid nitrogen to destroy precisely targeted skin cells. Following treatment, the skin naturally regenerates. Excess melanin rises to the surface and, after a few days, flakes off. How well this works depends on how deep the pigment lies. Freckles can also be treated with cryotherapy.

TOPICAL AGENTS FOR SKIN DISCOLORATION

Topical lightening formulations can be combined with other treatments to help reduce skin pigmentation. They do their work by inhibiting enzymes that produce melanin (skin pigment) or by increasing the turnover of the skin, to flush out existing pigmentation. Common lightening agents include; hydroquinone, kojic acid, paper mulberry bark extract, retinoids, and glycolic acid.

Read more about skin lightening creams in our section under 'Skin Therapy' (page 184).

SKIN ISSUES: DRY SKIN

Dry skin (also called *xerosis*), is a common condition that occurs in people of all ages. Generally it's not a serious problem but it can contribute to the appearance of lines and wrinkles, and make you look older than you really are. Dry skin is also more vulnerable to pathogens.

CAUSES OF DRY SKIN

In normal skin, the sebaceous glands—oil-producing glands—maintain a healthy level of natural skin oil called sebum. This lubricates the skin and keeps it hydrated by preventing excessive water loss or excessive water absorption. Normal skin has a supple feel and looks moist, but not greasy.

Hyaluronic acid is a natural substance distributed widely throughout our bodies, including our skin. It is involved in tissue repair and skin moisturization. The skin's content of hyaluronic acid decreases as the years pass.

The skin's natural barrier is an outer layer of fatty substances (lipids) that shields skin cells from harmful materials while allowing moisture and nutrients to enter. Dry skin occurs when the lipid barrier becomes damaged. When skin cells are exposed, they lose water to the atmosphere, and the skin's appearance deteriorates. The effect is made worse if there is also a decrease in sebum production.

PROTECTING THE SKIN'S NATURAL BARRIER AND OILS

Avoid regular, harsh scrubbing

You do not necessarily need to scrub your skin with a brush, loofah or exfoliating gloves to get it clean. Friction strips the skin and enhances the dryness. Be gentle with your skin. Use your hands or a soft washcloth instead.

Take shorter, cooler baths and showers

Prolonged bathing in hot water can remove the natural oils from the skin. The longer you stay in the bath or shower, the more you dry out your skin. To guard against this problem bathe in lukewarm water rather than hot water, and keep your showers and baths short. Many people like to add bath oils to their bathwater.

Use soap-free cleansers

Washing with harsh soaps removes your skin's natural moisture barrier. Instead, use a mild, fragrance-free cleanser that moisturizes as it removes grime. Commercial products are available in the form of bars or liquids. If your skin is dry, select a product that is particularly designed for dry skin.

Home-made Skin Cleansers

Make your own soap-free cleansers at home. Visit our 'Recipes' section (page 250).

Use moisturizer after bathing

When you take a shower, your epidermis absorbs some water and after the shower your skin will be covered with moisture. Rubbing yourself dry with a towel straight afterwards strips away that moisture, and any water that was absorbed by the skin will be lost to evaporation if you do not seal it in.

It is not only the skin on your face that needs hydration, but the skin on your body too. To seal in moisture and add extra, apply a deep-moisturizing cream or body-lotion all over the body. Choose products with rich, emollient ingredients such as shea butter, cocoa butter, or jojoba oil. Scrubbing your body with exfoliating gloves while showering will remove dead skin cells and allow the after-shower lotion to penetrate more easily.

Home-made Moisturizers

Make your own skin moisturizers at home. Visit our 'Recipes' section (page 250).

Increase humidity when temperatures are very high or low

In cold weather, when the temperature drops, so does the air's humidity level. Parched air dries out the skin. Turning up indoor heating does not fix the problem because high temperatures drive even more moisture from the air, and therefore from your skin.

To solve this problem, install a humidifier in your home to keep air moist. Set humidity at a constant 45% to 55%, and the temperature to around 20 degrees Celsius (68 degrees Fahrenheit). When going outdoors, apply a moisture barrier cream or ointment to your lips and face. Protect your neck and hands with a scarf and gloves.

ADDING MOISTURE TO THE SKIN

Combat aging with hyaluronic acid

Hyaluronic acid exists as a 'filling material' in most of our connective tissues—especially the skin. It protects the skin, stabilizes the skin's structure and provides elasticity.

As the skin on your face, your neck, your décolletage and your hands loses hyaluronic acid and dries out, it becomes susceptible to the formation of wrinkles and lines. Good skin hydration is essential to your well-being and appearance.

Hyaluronic acid acts as a skin hydrating agent when injected by a skilled technician. Hydration injectable therapy involves micro injections of this substance to boost your skin's moisture and suppleness from within. Learn more in our section on hydrating dermal fillers (page 160).

Use skincare products containing ammonium lactate and urea

Ammonium lactate is a moisturizer. Urea loosens thick or scaly skin cells and allows them to shed. The combination of ammonium lactate and urea, applied to the skin, is used to treat rough or scaly skin caused by such conditions as eczema or psoriasis. This formulation will also help soften cracked skin or calluses. Protect the skin from sunlight and do not use ammonium lactate on the face.

Drink sufficient water

Most of the moisture in your skin is supplied by the water you drink. It is recommended that you drink around seven to eight glasses of water every day (you can drink it in the form of herbal or green tea, if you wish) to ensure your skin stays well hydrated.

Exfoliate - but not too much

Scrubbing is fine, and even desirable, as long as it is not too frequent or too harsh. In fact, a regular once-a-week scrub is a great way to exfoliate (i.e. remove dead skin cells from your face and body), so that your moisturizers and serums can sink in and do their job. Never rub too hard or exfoliate more than about twice a week at the most, or you will damage your skin's natural barrier and end up with dry skin.

NOURISHING YOUR SKIN

Choose a healthy diet and lifestyle

A balanced diet of fresh, wholesome food is the best way to keep your skin healthy. Feed your body with all the vitamins, minerals and fatty acids to help your skin stay hydrated.

Lifestyle habits that can harm and dry out your skin include smoking, drinking alcohol in excess, and consuming large amounts of caffeine (e.g. in coffee, chocolate or soft drinks). As time passes the cumulative effects of these habits will show up as wrinkles and sagging skin.

Use a vitamin C serum

Choose skincare products that contain Vitamin C, if possible. This powerful antioxidant not only protects your skin from harmful environmental factors, it also encourages collagen production. With enough collagen, your skin will stay plump and elastic, locking in its own moisture for its freshest, healthiest look possible.

Home-made Vitamin C Serum

Make your own vitamin C serum at home. Visit our 'Recipes' section (page 250).

Use a vitamin A serum

Skin that lacks vitamin A (retinol) can become scaly and dry. Choose skincare products contain that retinol–a form of vitamin A– and apply them at night. Retinol can make your skin sun-sensitive, so wear sunscreen during the day. Tretinoin (the carboxylic acid form of vitamin A) is considered the best topical therapy for improving fine facial wrinkles, but it is available only on prescription.

Home-made Vitamin A Serum

Make your own vitamin A serum at home. Visit our "Recipes" section (page 250).

Balance your hormones

Dry skin can be caused by hormone imbalances. Hormone levels are influenced by factors such as nutrition, diet, lifestyle, exercise, stress, emotions, age and ovulation.

If you think you are suffering from a hormonal imbalance, consult your doctor. It is important to obtain a professional diagnosis and medical advice on treatment options.

A nutritious, balanced diet is crucial to promote normal hormone levels. Avoid processed foods – particularly refined sugars. A diet that includes wholegrains, nuts, seeds, fruits and vegetables will maintain good health and help regulate hormone production.

Avoid over-exposure to sunlight

Limiting your skins exposure to damaging environmental factors can do much to improve its health and keep it hydrated. The skin's moisture levels can be harmed by extreme heat or cold, but it is generally the ultraviolet (UV) rays in sunlight that cause the most damage. UV damage is cumulative.

Even small amounts of solar radiation penetrating the skin day by day can, over time, wreak havoc with your moisture levels. Protect your skin from the sun by using sunscreens and appropriate clothing.

Protect it, too, from wind, heat, cold and air pollution.

Be aware of your skin type
Is your skin dry or oily?

Dry skin can appear like oily skin. Skin can take on an 'oily' look when affected by hormones, excessive dryness, poor diet or emotional stress. This shiny or greasy look occurs when sebaceous glands produce more sebum than normal. Many cases of 'oily skin' are really instances of dry skin, which the skin tries to fix by increasing sebum production.

Both oily skin and dry skin often arise from many of the same basic causes. You might assume that the best remedy for this oily appearance is a decrease in hydration–for example by using de-greasing products on your skin every day in combination with scrubs and/or peels (which strip away the skin's lipid barrier) followed by 'lightweight' skin moisturizers.

This approach, however, can do more harm than good. Your aim should not be to replace the skin's natural hydration process, but to regain its natural balance. Moisturizers, cleansers and other skin care products used together can correct the cause of the oily appearance and return the skin to a more normal state.

Sensitive skin

Sensitive, allergic or 'reactive' skin responds adversely to even minor irritants by producing redness, inflammation, hives and/or pimple breakouts. Sensitive skin may be a result of a diamine oxidase enzyme deficiency, which causes histamine intolerance. It may also arise from nutritional deficiencies, mental stress or skin injury.

Learn more about histamine intolerance at www.low-histamine. com or read the book, *'Is Food Making You Sick? The Strictly Low Histamine Diet'*.

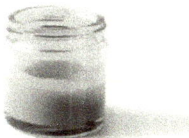

SKIN HYDRATION VS. SKIN MOISTURIZATION

Skin moisturization

The purpose of applying a moisturizer is to create a barrier to stop water loss from the skin. With this artificial barrier in place, it is easier for the body to repair its own natural barrier. Any gentle topical compound that creates a barrier between our skin and the world can be considered a moisturizer. Examples include mineral oil, jojoba oil and olive oil.

However, most commercial moisturizers contain much more than a simple barrier agent. These extra ingredients can smooth the skin, make it feel more flexible, speed up barrier repair, reduce inflammation, nourish the skin and so on. Such ingredients may include evening primrose oil, green tea extract, aloe vera and shea butter.

Evening primrose oil contains gamma-linoleic acid (GLA), an anti-inflammatory agent and barrier repair helper. It also contains phytosterols, polyphenols, vitamins, minerals, and other compounds to nourish the skin. Borage oil also contains GLA. Green tea extract contains polyphenols and anti-oxidants. Aloe vera can soothe damaged skin. Shea butter creates a barrier, but also includes fatty acids that soften the skin. Sunflower, soybean, and rice bran oil are all high in linoleic acid, a beneficial skin nutrient.

Moisturizers generally contain the following:

Occlusives – These create a hydrophobic (water repellent) barrier to reduce loss of water from the skin into the atmosphere. There are three barrier ingredients approved and recognized by the USA's Food and Drug Administration (FDA) –

- dimethicone
- cocoa butter
- allantoin

Other ingredients can be occlusive, but they are not FDA-approved barrier ingredients. There is some controversy about the safety of dimethicone, which is a silicone-based polymer.

Emollients – These moisturizer ingredients include oils, butters, and esters. They enhance the flexibility and softness of skin and provide a secondary soothing effect to the skin and mucous membranes. Emollients make our skin feel smooth.

Skin hydration

Hydration is defined as an adequate measure of water in our skin. It can be anywhere between 20% to 30% in the skin's top layer, the epidermis. Hydrating compounds generally contain humectants.

Humectants – these are compounds that draw water from the atmosphere and bind it, keeping it in the skincare product and thus on the skin. Examples of humectants include aloe vera, honey and glycerin.

Combining skin moisturization and skin hydration

Blending humectants, emollients and occlusives creates a skin care product that draws water to your skin, traps it, and makes the skin feel smooth and elastic.

If you have really dry skin and wonder why your daily application of an occlusive barrier product isn't helping your skin get any less dry, it's because you are not adding any moisture. The occlusive barrier ensures that you do not lose any more water, but it is not adding moisture to your skin.

To fix this problem, apply the occlusive barrier product over damp skin to create a layer of protected moisture. Over this layer, you can apply your humectants and emollients.

SKIN ISSUES: ECZEMA AND PSORIASIS

ECZEMA

Eczema, also known as atopic dermatitis, is an inherited, chronic skin condition that usually appears in early childhood. Patches of skin become red, dry, thickened and itchy, and may weep. Eczema is not contagious. There is no cure, but it can be managed. Some people 'outgrow' the condition.

TYPES OF ECZEMA

There are many different forms of eczema besides the most common form, atopic dermatitis. Others include:

- Contact dermatitis. There are two types of contact dermatitis—irritant contact dermatitis and allergic contact dermatitis. *Allergic contact dermatitis* is a reaction that occurs after the skin has come into contact with a substance that the body's immune system identifies as foreign. *Irritant contact dermatitis* is a localized reaction that occurs after the skin has come into contact with an allergen.
- Dyshidriotic eczema–irritation of skin on palms of hands and soles of feet, characterized by blisters.
- Neurodermatitis–scaly patches of skin on head, forearms, wrists, lower legs caused by localized irritants such as insect bites.
- Nummular eczema–circular patches of irritated skin that can be crusted, scaling and itchy.
- Seborrheic eczema–oily, scaly yellowish patches of skin, generally on the scalp and face.
- Stasis dermatitis–skin irritation on the lower legs, generally related to circulatory problems.[27]

---

27   *Source: www.medicalnewstoday.com.*

ECZEMA TRIGGERS

The specific cause of eczema is unknown, but it is thought to be a combination of hereditary and environmental factors. Environmental factors that can trigger the symptoms of eczema include:

- Irritants such as detergents, shampoos, soaps, and plant juices.
- Histamine intolerance (see www.low-histamine.com).
- Allergens including dust mites, pets, pollens, mold, and dandruff.
- Microbes: bacteria such as Staphylococcus aureus, viruses, and certain fungi.
- Hot and cold temperatures: hot weather, high and low humidity, perspiration from exercise.
- Foods such as dairy products, eggs, nuts and seeds, soy products, wheat.
- Emotional stress is not a cause of eczema but can make symptoms worse.
- Hormones: women can experience worsening of eczema symptoms at times when their hormone levels are changing, for example during pregnancy and at certain points in their menstrual cycle.

NON-SURGICAL ECZEMA TREATMENTS

Ultraviolet radiation therapy (phototherapy)
Exposure to ultraviolet radiation can help reduce the symptoms of chronic eczema. Exposure under medical supervision can be carefully monitored with the use of specially designed 'cabinets'. The patient stands naked in the cabinet and fluorescent tubes emit ultraviolet radiation. A person with stubborn eczema may need up to 30 sessions. The risks of unsupervised ultraviolet radiation therapy can be the same as for sunbathing – faster aging of the skin and greater risk of skin cancer.

Learn more by reading the section on ultraviolet radiation therapy (page 248).

Low histamine diet
Some people have achieved relief from eczema symptoms by excluding histamine-rich foods from their diet. Learn more about histamine intolerance at www.low-histamine.com or read the book *'Is Food Making You Sick? The Strictly Low Histamine Diet'*.

Other non-surgical eczema treatments
Topical moisturizers, corticosteroids taken in pill form or applied topically to the skin, preparations containing ammonium lactate and urea, and other skin care prescriptions and products are among the other therapies for eczema. Your doctor can advise you.

PSORIASIS

Psoriasis occurs when a person's skin cells grow more rapidly than normal. The body naturally forms new skin cells every month, to replace older skin that flakes off. With psoriasis, the new skin cells are formed every few days, instead of every few weeks. Because of this fast growth, dead skin cells build up on the skin's surface, causing patches of scaly, bumpy, thick, red, dry, itchy and sometimes painful skin.

'Psoriasis is a common, chronic, relapsing/remitting, immune-mediated inflammatory skin disease characterized by red, scaly patches, papules, and plaques, which usually itch and/or flake. The skin lesions seen in psoriasis may vary in severity from minor localized patches to complete body coverage. The disease affects 2–4% of the general population.'[28]

Scientists do not fully understand the causes of psoriasis. It is not merely a skin condition, because it can adversely affect other parts of the body, both internal and external. Unlike eczema, psoriasis frequently affects the outer side of the joint. It often appears on finger-nails and toenails. Up to 30% of people with psoriasis may also suffer from inflammation of the joints (psoriatic arthritis).

It is not contagious. There is no cure for psoriasis, but with the right treatment it can be well controlled.

28　*Wikipedia: Psoriasis. Retrieved 19th September 2014*

Types of psoriasis

The five main types of psoriasis are plaque, guttate, inverse, pustular, and erythrodermic. Plaque psoriasis is the most common form. It usually shows up as patches of silvery-white, scaly build-ups of skin cells. These plaques often form on the skin of the elbows and knees, but they can appear on any area of the body including the hands, the soles of feet, the underarms and the scalp.

NON-SURGICAL PSORIASIS TREATMENTS

Psoriasis symptoms can be relieved by a range of treatments, some of which have to be prescribed by doctors.

Ultraviolet radiation therapy (phototherapy)

Exposure to ultraviolet radiation can help reduce the symptoms of psoriasis. Phototherapy is unable to cure psoriasis, although it can be very beneficial to the skin of many patients. Phototherapy is a second-line treatment, used when first-line topical treatments have proved unsuccessful.

Learn more by reading the section on ultraviolet radiation therapy under 'Skin Therapy,' page 248.

Low histamine diet

Many people have achieved relief from psoriasis symptoms by excluding histamine-rich or histamine-releasing foods from their diet. Learn more about histamine intolerance at www.low-histamine.com or read the book 'Is Food Making You Sick? The Strictly Low Histamine Diet'.

Other psoriasis treatments

Other therapies for psoriasis include topical moisturizers, cortico-steroids taken in pill form or applied topically to the skin, preparations containing ammonium lactate and urea, and other skin care prescriptions and products. Medications include methotrexate, neotigason, cyclosporin and calcipotriol. Consult your doctor about this issue.

SKIN ISSUES: ENLARGED PORES

Enlarged facial pores can mar your appearance. They give your skin an irregular texture and tone that detracts from the smooth, glowing look it had when you were younger. Large pores become more noticeable as we age, because the skin's reduced elasticity causes them to dilate.

There is no permanent solution for treating enlarged pores. Treatments can temporarily reduce pore size to make them less noticeable. Multiple treatments can prolong the results. These may include:

- chemical peels
- microdermabrasion
- non-laser light therapy
- laser therapy

Treatments *not* recommended for pore refining include dermal fillers and ablative laser skin resurfacing. Ablative lasers without a fractional element are far too aggressive for minimizing pore size.

You can prolong the results of refining enlarged pores by keeping sun exposure, smoking and emotional stress to a minimum. The results may last for a few months up to a year or more, depending on your lifestyle, skin condition and skin type.

LASER TREATMENTS FOR REFINING ENLARGED PORES

Lasers generally improve the texture of the skin by increasing collagen production. Lasers may refine large pores, but they are not a primary treatment.

Ablative laser skin resurfacing

Ablation is the removal of body tissue. Ablative lasers, which go by several different trade names, directly affect the surface of the skin by peeling off the top layer. Their action also stimulates collagen production below the surface. *Fractional* ablative CO_2 lasers split light into a sort of grid, so that not all of the skin is affected at one time. After treatment, the skin requires three to five days to recover.

Extreme caution should be used when treating large pores with a fractional ablative laser. In some cases, the laser can remove enough skin so that pores actually look bigger.

Trade names of treatment techniques include Active FX® and Carbon Blast Laser®. The Carbon Blast Laser system uses a laser in conjunction with a 'carbon lotion' which is applied to the skin before treatment. This technique is said to refine enlarged pores, reduce oil secretion, remove blackheads and make the skin look paler.

Non-ablative laser skin resurfacing

Fractional non-ablative lasers cause more limited damage to the skin's surface while still stimulating collagen production in the deeper layers. Like all fractional lasers they distribute energy in checkerboard-like fragments, so that not all skin is affected at once. Common side effects include redness, peeling, and blistering.

Trade names of some treatment techniques to reduce pore size include the Lux 1540 erbium laser, Fraxel Laser®, Pearl®, and Laser Genesis®.

MICRODERMABRASION FOR REFINING ENLARGED PORES

Like any other treatment, microdermabrasion cannot actually shrink pore size, but it can unplug pores that are clogged with dead skin cells and oils, thus making them appear smaller.

Microdermabrasion exfoliates the skin, getting rid of dead skin cells on the surface. In addition to minimizing the appearance of pores it can brighten skin and reduce the appearance of scars. It is also cheaper than most chemical and laser peels.

If you have sensitive skin which is too delicate for chemical peels and laser treatments, you might consider microdermabrasion.

NON-LASER LIGHT THERAPY FOR PORE REFINING
Isolaz®

Isolaz is the trade name of a device that combines intense pulsed light (IPL) therapy with vacuum suctioning to clean out large pores, removing bacteria, oils, and dead skin cells. Isolaz can be used on most parts of the body, including the face. The Isolaz technique is suitable for all skin types.

LED skin treatment

Light emitting diode (LED) therapy stimulates the skin's collagen production. Increased collagen promotes skin elasticity and better support for the walls of pores. Thus supported, pores appear to shrink. Of the available LEDs, red light is the most effective for treating oily or acne-prone skin, as it encourages cell turnover and reduces pore size. At least five sessions are needed before results become noticeable.

Photodynamic therapy (PDT)

Photodynamic therapy (PDT) treats enlarged pores clogged with oil. By destroying the bacteria and oils within the pores, PDT may reduce pore inflammation. Some methods use a combination of a light-activated formulation applied to the skin (either a liquid or a cream, depending on the brand) with the light source. PDT is recommended for use on light-colored skin.

CHEMICAL PEELS FOR REFINING ENLARGED PORES
Alpha Hydroxy Acid (AHA) peels

An AHA peel is a light chemical peel that removes a thin surface layer of skin and promotes cell growth. AHA peels can use a variety of chemicals to peel the skin, but glycolic acid is the optimal ingredient for reducing pore size.

AHA peels can contain from 30% up to 70% glycolic acid—the higher the concentration, the stronger the peel. Being water-soluble, AHAs are used to treat dry skin.

(🐷)**Home-made AHA Peel**
Make your own alpha hydroxy acid (AHA) peels at home. Visit our "Recipes" section (page 250).

Beta hydroxy acid (BHA) peels

BHA peels are a good treatment for large pores because the chemicals are lipid-soluble, meaning they are attracted to your skin's oils. This is why BHA peels are also good for oily complexions.

The main ingredient in BHA peels is salicylic acid, a natural ingredient that gently peels dead cells from the surface of the skin. In addition to this exfoliation, salicylic acid can unclog pores. These actions combine to make the pores look more refined. The best concentration for a BHA peel is 20% to 30% salicylic acid.

Enlarged pores cannot be entirely eliminated, and the results will not be permanent. Regular BHA peels are required to maintain the appearance of smaller pores.

(🐷)**Home-made BHA Peel**
Make your own beta hydroxy acid (BHA) peels at home. Visit our "Recipes" section (page 250).

Trichloroacetic acid (TCA) peels

The TCA (trichloroacetic acid) peel is a medium depth chemical peel that can reduce enlarged pores. TCA not only exfoliates, it also strengthens the skin's supporting structure by encouraging collagen growth.

TCA peels are strong, and can damage the skin if not formulated and used correctly, so we recommend visiting a professional esthetician or dermatologist if you wish to have a TCA peel.

Obagi (TM) 'Blue Peel'

Large pores can be treated with an Obagi® blue facial peel, manufactured by Obagi Systems.[29] The blue tint permits the TCA chemical solution to be applied in precisely measured layers. These peels are performed in-office by trained specialists. Seven to ten days after treatment, a smooth, more youthful skin layer with refined pores is revealed.

Jessner's peel

'Jessner's solution' is a peeling formulation composed of 14% resorcinol, 14% lactic acid and 14% salicylic acid in an alcohol base. It is a medium to deep strength peel, depending on the number of layers applied. A Jessner's peel is particularly effective for oily skin and acne problems. The salicylic acid deeply penetrates the skin and removes sebum and dead skin cells that are congesting the pores. Jessner's peels are sometimes used in conjunction with microdermabrasion for severe skin issues.

FACIALS FOR REFINING ENLARGED PORES

Facials can help reduce the appearance of enlarged pores. Pores expand naturally with age, as the skin loses elasticity, making it easier for dirt to get trapped inside. A facial is meant to remove unwanted oil and debris from within your pores, making them less obvious.

Many spas and beauty clinics also offer specialized facials meant to tighten the pores, using creams containing antioxidants or ingredients that boost collagen production. Examples include the 'green tea facial'.

PORE REFINING AT HOME

The pores on your face (particularly the nose) become enlarged when they are clogged with oil, sebum, dead skin cells and other detritus. People with thick, oily skin tend to develop large pores more

---

29   *Obagi products are cruelty-free and safe for vegans and vegetarians.*

often than people with normal or dry skin. Keeping your skin clean and moisturized will improve the condition.

Following a good skin care regimen will help to clear the pores and make them appear smaller. Learn how to cleanse your pores by reading our 'Step by step guide to blackhead and whitehead removal at home', page 56.

If your enlarged pores refuse to respond to your cleansing efforts, visit a dermatologist or trained esthetician who can provide professional exfoliation regimes, deep peels, or laser treatments to boost collagen and minimize the appearance of pores.

Home-made Pore Refining Masks
Make your own pore refining masks at home. Visit our "Recipes" section on page 250.

SKIN ISSUES: SCARS, STRETCH MARKS & POCK MARKS

Scars, stretch marks and pock marks can be treated with a variety of techniques involving lasers, light-emitting devices, radiofrequency, injections and medications.

SCARS
Scars are areas of fibrous tissue that replace normal skin after an injury has healed. A scar results from the process of wound repair in the skin and the deeper tissues of the body. It is a natural part of the healing process. With the exception of very minor scratches, every wound on the human body (for example, after accident, disease, or surgery) results in some degree of scarring.

Scar tissue is made of collagen, the same protein as the skin tissue that it replaces. The fiber composition of the protein is different in scars – instead of a random basket-weave formation of the collagen fibers occurring in normal tissue, in scars the collagen cross-links and aligns itself in a single direction.

This alignment of the scar collagen does not work as efficiently as the normal alignment. For instance, scarred skin is less resistant to the sun's ultraviolet radiation. Also sweat glands and hair follicles are unable to form within scar tissue.

There are no magical cures for permanently scarred skin, but there are some treatments which may reduce the red or brown discoloration, or soften the thickening of scar tissue.

TYPES OF SCARS AND THEIR TREATMENTS

Red scars

Most scars will be red during the healing phase and in most cases this will fade spontaneously. Persistent redness in scars may respond to Pulsed Dye Laser treatment (page 210). Pulsed Dye Laser is also used to remove reddish blood vessel blemishes and birthmarks.

Brown scars

Some people may develop brown discoloration in patches of damaged skin. Generally this fades naturally over time, but if it persists for longer than nine months, it can be treated with a Q-Switched YAG laser or the minimally ablative Q-switched Ruby laser to help fade the pigmentation. See "Skin Therapy: laser skin therapies" on page 206.

Treatment with a prescription skin lightening cream such as hydroquinone 4% may also be useful. See page 233.

Raised (hypertrophic) scars

In rare cases scar tissue may over-develop, causing thickened, raised tissue. This is known as hypertrophic scarring. In some people this skin reaction is so extreme that even a scratched insect bite can result in a thick scar.

Generally, hypertrophic scarring will resolve naturally over a period of about twelve months. Treatment can speed up this process and for people in whom the scarring does not resolve, treatment can also help. People who have a tendency to this form of 'over healing' are usually aware of the problem, and if they tackle it early they will get the best results.

After finding out the patient's medical history and inspecting other scars, a dermatologist or cosmetic technician can counteract the overgrowth of scar tissue with regular micro-injections of cortisone solution. If the problem is not addressed until after the scar has formed, the tissue may still respond to micro-injection treatment.

You can also buy, from pharmacies and drug stores, silicone sheeting designed to flatten raised scars.

Keloid scars

Keloid scars are a more severe problem and the tendency is often genetic. It is more common in darker skin types. The classic feature of keloid scarring is that it grows and invades beyond the site of the actual injury. It is also often extremely sensitive and prone to itching. Keloid scarring commonly occurs in acne lesions on the chest and back.

Treatment for keloid scarring is similar to that described for hypertrophic scarring. This condition also has the tendency to recur over the years and require repeated courses of treatment. People prone to keloid scarring should consider preventative treatment as early as possible following injury. They should also avoid unnecessary surgery.

Stretch Marks

As discussed earlier, there are three layers to the skin: the epidermis (outer layer), dermis (middle layer) and hypodermis (deepest layer). Stretch marks develop in the middle layer. When the dermis is stretched or otherwise damaged it becomes less elastic, resulting in dark colored stretch marks. Over time these marks become pale in color and sink below the level of the rest of the skin.

Stretch marks are often the result of the rapid stretching of the skin associated with swift growth (common in puberty) or weight gain (e.g. pregnancy, muscle building, or fast gaining of fat). Although stretch marks are unsightly, they pose no health problem.

Treatment of stretch marks

Treatment involves fading the color, strengthening the collagen and developing new youthful collagen. Stretch marks will not disappear completely but their appearance can be vastly improved. The type of treatment depends on the types of stretch marks–red, white, old or new–and where on the body the stretch marks are placed.

Stretch marks can be treated with a series of sessions with lasers or radiofrequency devices. Treatment programs usually requires 3–5 session 4–6 weeks apart.

Fractional lasers such as the 1540 Fraxel Laser are well-suited for the task. Treatment with this device reduces the pigmentation of stretch marks. It can also stimulate new collagen production and tighten existing older collagen.

Radiofrequency skin therapy is said to result in more than 50% improvement. It delivers heat deep into the dermis without damaging to the shallower layers. The technique tightens collagen and stimulates growth of new and younger collagen. This process rejuvenates and firms the surrounding skin while reducing stretch marks.

Pock Marks

'Pock mark' may refer to:
- Acne scarring–resulting from acne or infections such as chicken pox.
- The scarring caused by smallpox.

For information on the different types of pock marks and their treatments, see our section on 'Acne and Acne Scarring', page 47.

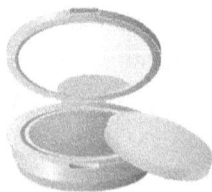

SKIN ISSUES: SKIN LAXITY

Genetics, sun exposure, and collagen and elastin degeneration cause our skin to sag as we age. The collagen that supports the skin breaks down, and areas that were once taut (e.g. knees, upper arms, stomach) start to look baggy. Collagen loss also makes cellulite more apparent because the skin becomes thinner and less able to conceal the puckers created by the superficial fat and connective tissue just below its surface. There is no topical remedy.

DEEP SKIN TIGHTENING FOR THE BODY

Deep skin tightening for the body usually targets lax skin on the abdomen, back, arms and thighs. It is best achieved by cosmetic surgery. Patients who do not feel ready for cosmetic surgery have a number of laser, radiofrequency and infrared options for deep skin tightening. Learn more by reading the section on deep skin tightening for the body in the companion book *'Beauty: The Ultimate Cosmetic Guide. Book 2: Body, Teeth and Hair'*.

SKIN TIGHTENING FOR THE FACE

Facelift

Surgical procedures such as facelifts, eyelid skin reduction (blepharoplasty) and brow lifts can elevate and tighten facial skin.

For people with skin laxity around the jawline, a lower facelift offers the most dramatic results. It also requires general anesthesia and weeks of downtime, and leaves scars around the earlobes.

Not everyone feels comfortable with the idea of surgery. With new technology and techniques, it is now possible to lift and tighten the face without surgery. These techniques are minimally invasive, and usually require no significant recovery period. Naturally the results are not as impressive as the results of surgery.

Learn more about facelifts by reading our section on facelift surgery, under 'Face Therapy' (page 130).

Thread lifts

Thread lifts can improve skin elasticity by boosting collagen production. They are a minimally-surgical method of lifting the tissues of the face by using specialized suture material. These sutures are inserted beneath the skin with a fine needle. Because they are lined with small barbs, they are able to grab on to the skin and hold it in a higher position. Learn more by reading the section on thread lifting under 'Face Therapy' (page 140).

Microneedle radiofrequency

Microneedle radiofrequency is used to treat facial skin laxity. Electrodes inserted beneath the skin conduct radiofrequency energy into the dermis, triggering collagen and elastin synthesis. The process is painful, so the doctor injects a local anesthetic to numb the face. After the treatment the patient usually experiences swelling, redness and perhaps some bruising. This resolves in about a week. Practitioners of this technique say that the results can last for several years. Trade names of microneedle radiofrequency devices include Miratone®.

Learn more about radiofrequency and skin needling by reading the relevant sections under 'Skin Therapy' (page 184).

Microneedling

The technique, also known as 'skin needling,' involves rolling a special device over the treatment area. In some devices the needles jut from a cylindrical roller; in others they are attached to a 'wand' or 'pen'. Numerous tiny needles puncture the skin many times, causing thousands of microscopic injuries. This stimulates the growth of collagen which, over time, improves the appearance of fine wrinkles and certain scars.

Microneedling is not generally considered to be the best way to tighten skin—it is more useful for improving the look of scars, stretch marks and uneven skin texture. Read more on page 238.

Radiofrequency

Radiofrequency (RF) devices are used to improve the appearance of both skin laxity and cellulite. Radiofrequency energy heats the collagen below the skin's surface, causing it to contract. Over time, the skin becomes tighter and firmer. Large areas such as the stomach and thighs can be treated.

Because radiofrequency works by heating collagen, patients must have sufficient collagen to begin with. This technique is most effective on skin that is mildly to moderately lax. Skin that is severely loose receives little to no benefit. Improved skin tightness may last for up to three years, while improvement in the appearance of cellulite generally lasts six to twelve months.

Trade name Thermage®: Thermage treatment can be somewhat painful, although taking a prescription-strength pain reliever can help. A single treatment session can produce improved tightness in the skin–not immediately, but after about three to six months, when new collagen has developed. No downtime is required.

Trade name Accent®: Like Thermage, this radiofrequency device can also tighten skin and improve the appearance of cellulite. It requires multiple treatments but causes much less discomfort than Thermage. No pain medication or downtime is required.

Trade name Pelleve®: Pelleve is said to be a relaxing and pleasurable treatment that gently heats the skin to a temperature at which the collagen fibers shrink and cause the skin (over the next few weeks and months) to tighten. No pain medication or downtime is required.

Learn more by reading the section on radiofrequency skin therapy under 'Skin Therapy' (page 184).

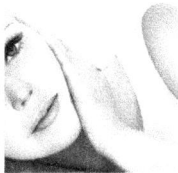

Fractional ablative laser treatment
Fractional ablative laser treatment is suited to patients over 55 years of age who have discolored, sun-damaged skin. This technique, which removes part of the top layer of skin cells, encourages the skin's production of new collagen, which not only tightens the skin but also improves its tone and texture.

Learn more about this technique in the section on laser skin therapies, under 'Skin Therapy' (page 206).

Non-ablative laser treatment
Non-ablative lasers deliver heat to the skin's surface to stimulate collagen growth and help improve skin tightness. It takes about three sessions to obtain results that compare to those of say, a single microneedle radiofrequency session; however the advantages include no pain and no downtime. It takes about six months for new collagen to completely finish forming and show maximum results. Eventually the improvement will start to wear off, unless it is maintained with regular treatments. Learn more by reading the section on laser skin therapies, under 'Skin Therapy' (page 206).

Infrared light
Infrared light therapy delivers sustained heat deep into the skin. It can tighten loose skin on the face, the area beneath the chin, the neck, the décolletage and the abdomen. Learn more in our section on infrared lasers under 'Skin Therapy' (page 211).

Trade names of infrared light devices include Cutera Titan®.

Ultrasound
The heat and vibrations delivered by ultrasound waves can heat the layers of skin and deeper tissues. One effect is to increase blood flow, helping the skin to regenerate. Another effect of ultrasound waves is to selectively injure the skin, triggering a natural healing response.

New collagen grows, and the elastin fibers straighten. In combination, these effects bring about lifting, tightening and firming of the skin.

Ultrasound energy can also benefit the top layer of skin, exfoliating it, smoothing the texture and improving the evenness of skin color.

Trade names of ultrasound skin tightening systems include Ulthera®.

Dermal fillers

One of the most noticeable features of facial aging is loss of volume in the skin. As the underlying collagen decreases over time, the skin begins to sag—much as an inflatable beach ball sags if it loses some air. Replenishing lost volume can 'plump up' the face, tightening and lifting the skin. Injectable dermal fillers are a popular method of returning volume to the face. They can be injected into areas such as the cheeks, brow, jawline, and chin. Learn more by reading the section on volumizing dermal fillers under 'Face Therapy' (page 162).

Carbon dioxide laser resurfacing

The ablative CO2 laser is used to resurface skin for the reduction of wrinkles, sun damage, pigmentation problems, and also to tighten skin. It actually removes a layer of skin as well as heating the skin to tighten it.

This method is particularly effective for skin tightening around the eyes. It can be performed in fractional mode (small columns of laser energy are fired into the skin, leaving some untreated skin) which reduces healing times, or in non-fractional mode, which has greater downtime. Learn more in our section on laser skin therapies, page 206.

Sunscreen

Sunscreen cannot bring back lost skin elasticity. It can, however, help prevent the UV-induced collagen loss that will make skin look saggier and more dimpled, so wear it whenever you are outdoors, no matter whether the day is cloudy or sunny.

SKIN ISSUES: SKIN LESIONS

'A skin lesion is a superficial growth or patch of the skin that does not resemble the area surrounding it.'[30]

Skin lesions can look unattractive, or cause problems by rubbing against clothing. Most skin lesions are benign, but you should check with your doctor if you are worried that a lesion on your body may be cancerous. Cancerous lesions should be removed by a medical specialist.

SKIN LESIONS INCLUDE:

Acne

Acne occurs when skin pores become blocked by oil, bacteria, and dirt, leading to infection. Severe acne can be painful and may result in scarring.

Actinic Keratosis

Actinic keratosis, or sun spots, is a common skin condition. It occurs when skin cells grow abnormally, forming scaly, discolored spots.

Boils (furuncles)

Boils are deep, localized and painful skin infections that develop on hair follicles. Also known as 'furuncles' or 'abscesses', they usually begin as small, sore, reddened bumps on the skin, later developing a soft, pale, pus-filled center.

Bullae

Bullae are fluid-filled sacs or lesions that appear when fluid is trapped under a thin layer of skin. Similar to blisters, bullae are larger.

Cherry Angioma

Cherry angiomas are small, bright red skin growths that are circular or oval in shape. They can grown on most areas of the body.

---

30   *The Free Dictionary by Farlex.*

Cysts

A cyst is a sac-like pocket of tissue that contains fluid, air, or other substances. Cysts can grow almost anywhere in the body or on the skin.

Erysipelas

Erysipelas is a bacterial infection that affects the skin's upper layers and causes lesions. It most commonly affects the legs, but can also affect the face. It usually begins when the bacteria enter the skin by way of a scratch or other wound. A reddened area of skin develops and spreads rapidly. It may be accompanied by fever and headaches, and requires professional treatment.

Freckles

Freckles are discolored spots on the skin; clusters of concentrated melanin. Causes of freckles include genetics and exposure to the sun.

Keloids

Keloids are smooth, hard skin growths that sometimes form when scar tissue grows excessively. They are not harmful but may be large and unsightly.

Lentigines

A lentigo (plural: lentigines), as mentioned elsewhere in this book, is a spot on the skin that is darker (usually brown) than the surrounding skin. Lentigines are more common among people with fair skin.

Exposure to the sun is thought to be the major cause of lentigines. Lentigines most often appear on parts of the body that get the most sun, including the face and hands. Some lentigines may be caused by genetics (family history) or by medical procedures such as radiation therapy.

Lipomas

Lipomas are noncancerous growths of fatty tissue that develop just under the skin, typically appearing on the neck, shoulder, back, abdomen, arms, and thighs. They look like small, dome-shaped lumps.

Moles

Moles occur when cells in the skin grow in a cluster instead of being spread throughout the skin. These cells are called melanocytes, and they manufacture the pigment that gives skin its natural color. Moles may darken after exposure to the sun, during the teen years, and during pregnancy.

Molluscum Contagiosum

Molluscum contagiosum is a skin infection that is caused by the molluscum virus. It produces round, firm, benign and painless bumps on the upper layers of the skin.

Nodules

A nodule is an abnormal growth that forms under the skin, often filled with inflamed tissue or fluid. These skin lesions are harmless but can be confused with cysts, tumors, and abscesses.

Pock Marks

Also known as varicella, chickenpox is a virus that often affects children. It is characterized by itchy, red blisters that appear all over the body. These can leave indentations called pock marks. Other causes of pock marks include acne scarring and smallpox.

Scars

Scars can result from injuries such as burns and cuts. They are areas of fibrous tissue (fibrosis) that replace the normal skin.

Sebaceous Cysts

Sebaceous cysts are common, non-cancerous skin cysts, often found on the face, neck, or torso. They look like small, smooth, painless lumps under the skin, and are not life-threatening but may be uncomfortable.

Seborrheic Keratosis

Seborrheic keratosis is a type of harmless skin growth that bears a resemblance to skin cancer. The growths may have a rough, wart-like surface and a waxy look. Their appearance can vary widely, from smooth to rough, from pale to dark. Their size generally ranges from 0.2 – 3 cm. They have well-defined borders and look as if they are simply glued onto the skin.

Seborrheic keratoses are more common in older people. Their cause is unknown, and they usually appear on the head, neck, or torso. Seborrheic keratoses are non-cancerous (benign) although sometimes they can resemble melanomas because of their irregular borders. In some cases, keratoses cause itching or irritation.

These skin lesions can be removed with surgery, laser, freezing, or scraping. Vitamin D3 ointment is also being tested as a treatment.

Skin Tags

Skin tags are small, harmless growths, usually the same color as the skin or darker. They hang off the skin like a tiny pouch, often growing on neck, breasts, groin, stomach, eyelids, and underarms.

Stretch Marks

Stretch marks or striae (singular: 'stria'), as they are called in dermatology, are a form of discolored scarring on the skin. They are caused by tearing of the dermis. Over time stretch marks may diminish, but they will not disappear completely.

Stretch marks are usually the result of the skin being stretched quickly, due to swift growth, swift weight gain or pregnancy. They can also be associated with factors such as hormonal changes during puberty or hormone replacement therapy, or a rapid increase in muscle due to bodybuilding.

Warts

Warts are raised bumps on the skin caused by the human papillomavirus (HPV). They are generally not dangerous but are contagious and can be painful.

SKIN LESION REMOVAL METHODS:

Surgery
Many general practitioners perform minor surgery in their clinic for benign and small malignant skin lesions. *Radiowave skin surgery* is a unique, less invasive, and highly effective treatment for skin lesion removal–particularly the removal of benign skin lesions on the face or other parts of the body.

Radiofrequency Microneedling
Radiofrequency microneedling is used in the treatment of acne and to improve acne scarring. Learn more on page 231.

Cryosurgery
Cryosurgery is the process of destroying a non-melanoma skin lesion by freezing it with liquid nitrogen. The skin may first be numbed with a local anesthetic. Liquid nitrogen is applied to the lesion using a cotton applicator stick or an aerosol spray. The application may be repeated. The doctor may apply an antibiotic dressing to the wound.

Cryosurgery is often used to destroy precancerous skin lesions such as actinic keratoses, but is rarely used alone to treat skin cancer.

Chemical Peels
Chemical peels, in effect, strip the skin of precancerous cells, preventing the disease from taking hold. Many dermatologists prescribe the Jessner's peel, a very effective light-to-medium-strength peel that treats large areas of the face that have precancerous lesions. Patients typically receive a series of these peels over several months. Learn more on page 194.

Ultrasound Skin Therapy
Scar tissue and contracture can be greatly improved with ultrasound treatment. Learn more on page 244.

Dermabrasion and microdermabrasion
When the technique of dermabrasion was first developed, it was used primarily to improve acne, pock marks and scars resulting from accidents or disease. Today, it is used to treat other skin issues, such as tattoo removal, sun damage, age/liver spots and wrinkles. It is one of the most popular treatments for skin lesion removal. See page 202.

Infrared LED Skin Treatment
"Red light easily penetrates the dermis and can help with a variety of skin conditions, such as acne, rosacea, scarring and eczema, as well as improving skin quality," says Jo Martin, clinical director of Mapperley Park Clinic. Learn more on page 219

Intense Pulsed Light (IPL)
IPL photofacials are often used to treat precancerous skin lesions and heavy sun damage. Learn more on page 217.

Laser Skin Therapies
There are numerous types of cosmetic lasers, most of which are extremely effective at skin lesion removal. Learn more by reading "Skin Therapy: laser skin therapies" on page 206.

Photodynamic Therapy (PDT)
PDT is currently being used or investigated as a treatment for the following skin conditions:
- Actinic keratoses on the face and scalp
- Basal cell carcinomas
- Bowen's disease (squamous cell carcinoma in situ)
- Squamous cell carcinoma
- Mycosis fungoides (cutaneous T-cell lymphoma)
- Kaposi sarcoma
- Psoriasis
- Viral warts

Learn more about photodynamic therapy on page 224.

SKIN ISSUES: VARICOSE AND SPIDER VEINS

Treatments for varicose and spider veins include sclerotherapy, radiofrequency, laser ablation and surgery.

VARICOSE VEINS

Varicose veins look like knobbly, twisted and darkish-blue cables just beneath the skin. They are most commonly found on the legs. They are caused by faulty valves within veins that allow the blood to pool.

SPIDER VEINS

Spider veins, also known as thread veins, are smaller, more easily visible veins which are closer to the skin surface. They are mostly found on the legs or face. Long-term use of potent steroid creams may also cause spider veins. Factors that can increase your chance of developing spider veins include:

- spending a lot of time on your feet
- being overweight
- getting older
- having a family history of spider veins
- pregnancy
- taking the oral contraceptive pill or hormone replacement therapy (HRT)
- the face being exposed to the sun

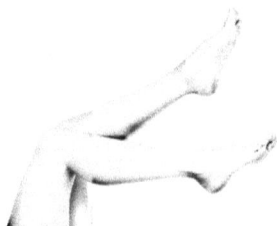

TREATMENTS FOR VARICOSE AND SPIDER VEINS

Surgery for varicose veins

Major surface veins that are varicose are usually treated surgically. Generally, a surgeon makes numerous small incisions (cuts) to reach the vein, rather than one large cut. Depending on the location of the varicose vein, these incisions may, for example, be in the groin or behind the knee.

Surgical techniques include:
- Ligation – the surgeon cuts and ties off the vein.
- Stripping – the surgeon makes a small cut in the vein, through which he or she inserts a narrow instrument. The vein is then pulled out through a second incision.
- Phlebectomy – the surgeon makes small incisions, then removes the veins with a special hook.

Sclerotherapy

With sclerotherapy, a medicine (sclerosant) is injected into the blood vessels, which makes them shrink. Sclerotherapy has been used in the treatment of varicose and spider veins and hemorrhoids for many years. Techniques have improved during that time, and now include methods like ultrasonographic guidance and foam sclerotherapy.

In ultrasound-guided sclerotherapy, (also known as 'echosclerotherapy') the physician uses ultrasound to 'see' the underlying vein. This enables the physician to deliver and monitor the injection more accurately.

Microsclerotherapy

Sclerotherapy was developed in the 1920s, but has since been refined for the treatment for spider/thread veins. The newer method is called 'microsclerotherapy'.

Foam Microsclerotherapy

Foam microsclerotherapy is the treatment of spider veins ('thread veins') using a sclerosant liquid or foam which is injected into the tiny veins, causing them to close. A very fine needle is used. The doctor generally uses a magnifying light to view the narrow blood vessels.

This is a particularly efficacious therapy for spider veins on the legs.

The sclerotherapy/microsclerotherapy procedure

The procedure takes a minimum of an hour and a half. Afterwards, the patient should walk around for about half an hour as part of the treatment. A typical sclerotherapy/microsclerotherapy treatment session follows this sequence:

• You stand up while the physician marks the site of injection on your legs.
• You lie down while the physician gives you the injections. The fine needle used for injecting does not cause much pain.
• As soon as you have had the injections, you put on compression bandages and stockings. The bandages fit tightly.
• While wearing these compression garments, you walk around for about half an hour.
• Many veins can be treated in one session. Each vein may need a number of injections, delivered several weeks apart. Allergic reactions are rare.

Radiofrequency

As discussed, the term 'ablation' refers to the use of heat to carefully damage body tissue. Radiofrequency ablation is a minimally invasive treatment for varicose veins. Radiofrequency energy is used instead of laser energy, to heat up and damage the wall inside a vein of the leg. The resulting scar tissue generally closes off the vein.

To treat a varicose vein with this method, the doctor inserts a thin tube – known as a 'catheter' – through a small incision in the vein. He or she then directs radiofrequency energy through this tube.

This technique can be used to treat large veins in the leg. It can be performed in the doctor's office using local anesthesia or a mild sedative. Patients are able to walk around soon after having the treatment, and recovery time is usually short.

After treatment, patients wear compression stockings for a week or more. To follow up, the doctor may use duplex ultrasound—a test to find out how blood flows through your arteries and veins—to ensure the vein is sealed off.

Electrodessication
With this treatment a high-frequency electric current is used to destroy tissue by dehydration, which seals the veins.

Laser ablation or other light therapy
Endovenous ablation is a minimally invasive treatment for varicose veins. The physician applies local anesthetic to the skin over the vein, then inserts a thin tube (catheter) into the vein. Through this catheter, laser energy is applied to the inside of the vein to seal it. Varicose veins may similarly be closed by the application of high-intensity light.

PREVENTION OF VARICOSE AND SPIDER VEINS

Some suggestions that may help to prevent varicose and spider veins include:

- Wearing support stockings.
- Maintaining a healthy weight.
- Exercising regularly.
- Avoiding wearing high heels, because they harm the correct functioning of the larger veins.

SKIN ISSUES: UNWANTED TATTOOS

Sometimes people get tattooed only to regret the decision later, for any number of reasons. Having an unwanted tattoo can be embarrassing and upsetting. It may also have social consequences, such as hampering one's ability to secure a job or a promotion.

If you don't want your tattoo to be seen any more you have three choices:

- conceal it with clothing or makeup,
- disguise it with a more acceptable tattoo,
- have it removed.

THE HISTORY OF UNWANTED TATTOOS

People have been tattooing each other for thousands of years—at least since Neolithic times. They have probably been wanting to remove some of these skin decorations since the Stone Age, too. Very early forms of tattoo removal included the injection or application of wine, lime, garlic or pigeon excrement.

Tattoo-removal experiments using short-pulsed lasers were first done in the late 1960s. Before the introduction of laser tattoo removal techniques however, common methods included:

- Dermabrasion.
- TCA (trichloroacetic acid, an substance that removes the layers of skin above the layer occupied by the tattoo ink).
- Salabrasion (scrubbing the skin with salt).
- Cryosurgery (freezing the tattooed skin with liquid nitrogen).
- Excision (this is sometimes still used in conjunction with skin grafts, to remove bigger tattoos).

LASER REMOVAL OF UNWANTED TATTOOS

These days, the most popular way to remove unwanted tattoos is by using lasers. The light emitted by non-invasive Q-switched laser devices can degrade the ink particles in the tattoo. The broken-down ink is then absorbed by the body, imitating the natural color-fading caused by aging or sun exposure.

All tattoo inks of varying colors have the ability to absorb varying parts of the light spectrum. Tattoo removal lasers emit the right amount of energy to be absorbed into each particular ink color.

Generally, black and darker-colored inks can be removed more completely. Certain tattoo pigments, such as yellows, greens and fluorescent inks are harder to treat than darker blacks and blues, because they absorb light waves that can't be easily emitted by tattoo removal lasers. An added problem is the recent introduction of pastel-colored tattoo inks that are rich in titanium dioxide, which is highly reflective. Such inks are difficult to remove because they reflect a lot of the laser's light energy out of the skin.

A number of different types of Q-switched lasers exist, and each is good at removing a different range of the color spectrum. Laser devices developed after the year 2006 are able to emit multiple wavelengths. This means they can treat a much broader range of tattoo pigments than earlier individual Q-switched lasers. The drawback with the wide-range pigment removal lasers, however, is that overall they may not be as efficient as using multiple separate specific wavelength lasers.

During the removal of unwanted tattoos by laser, pain relief is provided via a topical anesthetic and by cooling the area with a medical-grade chiller. The laser beam passes harmlessly through the skin layers, targeting only the liquid ink in the deeper layers. Sometimes the results are immediate, but usually the fading occurs gradually during the 7–8 week healing period between treatments.

Laser tattoo removal requires repeat visits.

Side effects may include some scarring and/or temporary changes in skin pigmentation. Areas with thin skin will be more likely to scar than thicker-skinned areas.

Rare risks include allergic reactions or ruptured blood vessels. Some tattoo pigments contain metals that could theoretically break down into toxic chemicals in the body when exposed to light. This has not yet been reported in vivo but has been shown in laboratory tests.[31]

Generally, your clinician will apply a topical anesthetic before laser removal of unwanted tattoos.

Learn more by reading the section on laser skin therapies (page 206).

SKIN ISSUES: WOUND HEALING

In the world of cosmetic therapy, faster and better wound healing is often achieved with the use of Low Level Laser Therapy (LLLT).

This treatment uses low-level lasers to boost the healing process at a cellular level. The effects of low-level laser therapy appear to be linked to the specific wavelength of the laser treatment itself.

Research demonstrates that the ideal wavelength, (dosage), duration and location of treatment is specific to each ailment and wound. The effective clinical dosage of low-level laser therapy for wound healing varies by manufacturer and remains a subject of continued research.

Learn more about Low Level Laser Therapy (LLLT) on page 219.

---

31   *Wikipedia 'Tattoo removal'. Article retrieved 12th October 2014.*

Part 3:
Face Therapy

FACE THERAPY

As we age our faces change. Skin loses its elasticity and begins to sag. Cheeks appear hollow and sagging jowls blur the once-crisp jawline. Foreheads droop. Wrinkles, lines and double chins may form.

There are many ways of correcting these issues, both surgical and non-surgical.

Some therapies to rejuvenate the appearance of the face include:

- Boosting collagen
- Brow lifting
- Cosmetic acupuncture
- Cosmetic tattooing (permanent makeup)
- Eyebrow treatments
- Facelift surgery
- Facial fat transfer
- Facial skin tightening
- Hydrating dermal fillers
- Jawline and neck rejuvenation
- Non-surgical facelifts
- Ribbon lifting
- Thread lifting
- Ultrasound face therapy
- Volumizing dermal fillers
- Wrinkle relaxing injections

The eyebrows, eyelashes and teeth all make an impact on the overall look of the face. In this book we discuss treatments for eyelashes and eyebrows, but we leave dental therapies—such as cosmetic dental contouring, teeth whitening and cosmetic gum reshaping—to the companion book in this series: 'Ultimate Beauty 2: Hair, Body and Smile.

FACE THERAPY: BOOSTING COLLAGEN

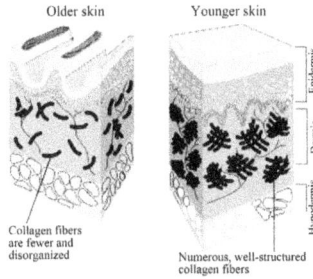

Older skin   Younger skin

Collagen fibers
are fewer and
disorganized

Numerous, well-structured
collagen fibers

Around 30% of the protein content of the human body is collagen. You can think of it as the 'glue' that holds the body together. Collagen is abundant in fibrous and connective tissues such as skin, ligaments and tendons. It is essential for strengthening our blood vessels and providing support and structure for various parts of our bodies. Collagen heals our skin, giving it firmness and some elasticity.

When our skin contains plenty of collagen it looks youthful. Along with elastin, collagen increases the 'springiness' of the skin's connective tissues, allowing them to expand and contract without damaging cells and causing wrinkles.

As we age, the production of collagen begins to slow down. Collagen loss is one of the major reasons or skin looks older as time passes. Our existing collagen degrades, and cell structures begin to lose their strength. Our skin becomes fragile, and less elastic. Wrinkles and other skin problems appear.

By the time we are in our thirties, collagen depletion overtakes collagen production. This is the time when we might begin to notice:

- Loss of volume in the cheeks, temples, lips and jawline.
- The development of lines and wrinkles, particularly in the folds between the nose and mouth.
- Sagging skin and the appearance of 'jowls' in place of your once-firm jawline.
- Dull, rough skin instead of the smoothness of youth.

Collagen boosting treatments are popular with older men and women.[32]

WAYS TO BOOST COLLAGEN

Laser Treatments

Laser treatments really do stimulate collagen production. Our skin contains fibroblasts, which are a type of cell that manufactures collagen and plays a vital role in wound healing. Laser skin treatments use light to break down our collagen. Collagen fragments then send signals to the fibroblasts, telling them to make a lot more collagen.

Some brand names of laser collagen-boosting treatments include V-Beam®, Thermage®, BBL®, Foto Facial®, Genesis®, and Clear and Brilliant®.

Intense Pulsed Light

Intense Pulsed Light (IPL) works the same way as laser therapy—by fragmenting collagen to encourage it to multiply.

IPL employs a broad wavelength light pulsed onto the skin. It can treat several conditions simultaneously, including

- Decreased collagen
- Broken veins and capillaries
- Redness of the skin
- Age spots, sun spots and freckles

Some brand names of IPL include Elos® and Limelight®.

Dermal Fillers

Injectable skin fillers can add volume to the skin, hydrate the skin or do both. They can correct fine lines, creases and folds and scars, and are also used for enhancing lips, reconstructing noses and chins, jawline sculpting and non-surgical rhinoplasty.

---

32   *Note: Evidence shows that eating collagen does not benefit your skin.*

Dermal fillers generally contain hyaluronic acid which, according to a study published in Archives of Dermatology, is thought to stimulate the production of collagen, restoring the structure of damaged skin. [33]

Unlike anti-wrinkle compounds such as Botox® and Dysport®, dermal fillers have no muscle-relaxing properties whatsoever.

Before you book an appointment to have dermal fillers injected, ask your clinician what areas he or she specializes in. Some treatments, such as nose or chin reconstructions, jawline sculpting and non-surgical rhinoplasty, should be done by a specialist.

Pain is minimal with this procedure, because an anesthetic cream will be applied to the area being treated, or you might receive a local anesthetic injection.

After treatment you may experience a few side effects such as minor redness, bruising and swelling, which usually resolve by themselves within 24 hours. Doctors will not inject dermal fillers into pregnant or nursing mothers, or people with a skin disease in the area to be treated.

Results usually last from 4 to 12 months, depending on the filler, the technique and the area that was injected. The more treatments you have, the longer the results will last.

Some brand names of dermal fillers include Restylane®, Radiesse® and Juvederm®.

Learn more by visiting the sections on volumizing dermal fillers (page 162) and hydrating dermal fillers (page 160).

Collagen Stimulating Injections
This technique involves the injection of a plant-derived substance called 'polylactic acid' (PLA), the same substance used by surgeons in dissolvable stitches.

---

33   *In vivo stimulation of de novo collagen production caused by cross linked hyaluronic acid dermal filler injections in photodamaged human skin. Archives of dermatology, 2007. Wang, Frank; Garza, Luis A; Kang, Sewon; Varani, James; Orringer, Jeffrey S; Fisher, Gary J; Voorhees, John J. Department of Dermatology, University of Michigan Medical School, Ann Arbor, MI 48109, USA. PMID: 17309996.*

A qualified practitioner uses a needle to deliver this substance into lines, wrinkles and depressions in the skin. Polylactic acid acts as a dermal filler, plumping up the skin's volume, while simultaneously helping to stimulate the body's own production of collagen.

Collagen stimulating injections can add volume to areas of the face and body that have become sunken or 'baggy'. They can be used to treat:

- lines and wrinkles on all parts of the face
- the forehead
- around the eye, especially 'tear troughs'
- around the lips
- between the mouth and nose
- the cheeks
- the neck
- the décolletage
- hands, knees and ankles
- certain types of scars

In general, a minimum of two sessions at least 15 days apart will give good results. Some estheticians recommend 3—4 treatments.

Improvement can be seen immediately following treatment. The full effect will appear about 20 days later. Due to polylactic acid's action of collagen stimulation, the results can last a lot longer than for other types of dermal fillers. Improvement can last from at least a year up to two years. Eventually the body will absorb the polylactic acid.

Brand names of collagen stimulating injections using polylactic acid include Sculptra™.

Gold threads

This is not a 'lift' in the sense of raising the skin tissues. Rather, it is a method of increasing collagen production in the face.

Using a needle, the doctor implants extremely fine, surgical-grade gold threads into the deeper skin layers. The gold triggers a biological response, and the skin begins to coat the threads with collagen.

Blood circulation increases in the surrounding tissue, supplying extra oxygen and nutrients. The skin begins to tighten and become more elastic, making the face appear more youthful.

SECRETS OF PRESERVING YOUR NATURAL COLLAGEN

To save and protect your own natural collagen, particularly in the face:

- Wear a good sun screen whenever you are outdoors.
- Avoid sun exposure between 10am and 3pm.
- Wear sunglasses to preserve the delicate skin around the eyes.
- Do not smoke.
- Avoid pollution.
- Apply skin creams containing Retin-A (tretinoin). Retin-A is a form of vitamin A that aids in skin renewal.
- Apply skin creams containing alpha-hydroxy acids, especially glycolic acid.
- Eat fresh fruits and vegetables.
- Cultivate good sleeping habits.

Some dermatologists also recommend taking antioxidants and anti-inflammatory agents such as resveratrol (a compound found largely in the skins of red grapes), acai, green tea, vitamin C (ascorbyl palmitate), Nicomide®, Coffeeberry®, and Pynogenol®.

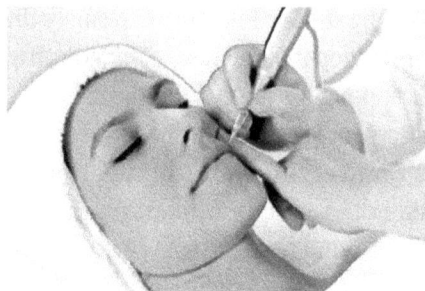

FACE THERAPY: BROW LIFTING

SURGICAL BROW LIFTING

Surgical brow lifting, sometimes known as forehead lifting, is a procedure that minimizes wrinkles and eye lines by raising the muscles and tissue of the area above the eyebrows.

Stress, sun exposure, smoking, poor nutrition and aging can all contribute to loss of skin elasticity, causing wrinkles and lines. Drooping eyebrows and furrows and creases in the forehead can make people appear tired, sad, angry or older than they actually are. Brow lifting can help rejuvenate your face.

Cosmetic surgeons frequently perform brow lifts in conjunction with other facial rejuvenation surgery such as an eyelid lift (blepharoplasty). It is sometimes suggested that patients who wish to undergo any cosmetic facial surgery should bear in mind the accompanying recovery time, and consider a combination of procedures to make the most of their time 'off work'.

To visualize the way you would look after brow lifting, place your hands on your temples (above your eyebrows, near the outside of your eyes) and gently and pull the skin upwards.

Surgical approaches

Multiple surgical approaches to brow lifting have been developed, and more than one may be used in combination by surgeons wishing to elevate the forehead skin.

Direct Brow Lift is performed by removing a segment of skin and muscle just above the eyebrows. This technique does not address wrinkles or lines within the forehead and surgical scars, despite being hidden within the eyebrow hair, may be prominent. It is typically reserved for older patients or for men with thick eyebrow hair and male pattern baldness for whom other techniques might result in unacceptable elevation of the hairline.

Mid-forehead Lift is intended for patients who have heavy sagging eyebrows and deeper forehead wrinkles. The surgeon makes incisions within the deep forehead wrinkles and removes the excess skin, fat and sometimes muscle. The resulting scars are concealed within the skin creases and are not very noticeable after healing. The advantage of this technique is that less of the forehead tissues need to be surgically loosened to elevate the eyebrows, and less skin needs to be removed when a site is chosen within the creases in the lower part of the forehead. Because this technique does not require elevating the skin of the whole forehead, the position of the hairline is not affected. This is advantageous for patients with high hairlines for whom more lifting of the hairline would be undesirable.

Coronal Brow Lift

This method involves a single incision, starting at one ear and finishing at the other, crossing the forehead slightly behind the hairline. The surgeon lifts the muscle and tissue of the forehead and removes excess skin and fat, before closing the incision with stitches.

Endoscopic Brow Lift

An endoscope is a thin instrument with a tiny camera at one end. The endoscope permits the surgeon to make minimal incisions while clearly viewing the treated area. Generally, the surgeon will make approximately five small incisions just behind the hairline, allowing him or her to insert surgical instruments beneath the skin to tighten and lift muscles and tissue. This method is much less invasive than the traditional 'coronal' method, and generally results in decreased recovery time and less scarring.

After a surgical brow-lifting procedure

The brow lifting procedure generally takes between one and two hours, depending on which surgical technique is employed. Usually, it can be done in the surgeon's rooms instead of requiring hospitalization, and the patient can return home after the effects of the anesthetic have worn off. However, the surgeon may recommend that the patient stays in hospital overnight.

After surgery the patient's head is wrapped in a bandage. This is removed within two days. Depending on the type of surgery, whether coronal lift or endoscopy, stitches can be removed within seven to fourteen days.

A couple of days after the procedure, patients should be able to undertake most of their usual daily activities, aside from of bending down and vigorous exercise. It is essential that patients abide by their surgeon's instructions and refrain from strenuous activity.

For up to ten days afterwards, patients will experience swelling and bruising in the forehead area and perhaps also the cheek and eye area.

The final results of brow lifting may take several weeks to a month to become obvious.

Potential risks and complications

As with any surgery, brow lifting can involve risks. Before you choose to undergo this procedure you ought to make sure you know all about these and discuss them with your surgeon.

Choose a fully qualified surgeon with accredited training in brow lift surgery who is experienced in the procedure.

Complications that may follow a brow lift include the possibility of permanent hair loss around the scar area on the scalp. This problem can be addressed with hair transplant surgery.

Some people experience immobility of muscles in the eyebrows or forehead after surgery. If this should occur, corrective surgery may be required.

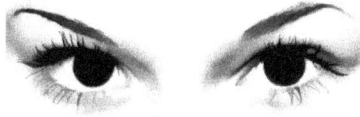

MINIMALLY INVASIVE BROW LIFTING (INCLUDING THE EYE AREA)

Dermal fillers (e.g. Restylane, Juvederm, Radiesse) can be used to lift the brow area. Clinicians can use them in conjunction with anti-wrinkle injections to can increase the distance between the eyebrow and the eyes.

This non-surgical brow lift can arch the eyebrow and give you a more youthful appearance. Learn more in the section about dermal fillers, page 162.

Wrinkle paralysis injections, also called anti-wrinkle injections or muscle-relaxing injections (e.g. Botox, Dysport, Xeomin), can also cause the brow area to appear lifted, especially is used in conjunction with dermal fillers. See page 183.

Platelet rich plasma injections (PRP) can be used in conjunction with fractional CO_2 laser therapy to enhance healing and improve results. These injections can plump up wrinkles, tighten the skin, lift sagging eyelids and improve the appearance of the eyes. See page 228 for more information.

NON-SURGICAL BROW LIFTING (INCLUDING THE EYE AREA)

Laser skin therapies: The newest and most advanced fractional CO_2 lasers can treat the wrinkles and aged skin around the eyes.

The fractional CO_2 laser uses modulated beams of light to penetrate and stimulate the collagen and elastin around the eyes. See also page 206.

FACE THERAPY: COSMETIC ACUPUNCTURE

Acupuncturists claim that the skilled use of acupuncture needles can 'remove blockages in the free flow of energy' on the hands, feet, scalp and face, and can help to firm the skin and reduce the appearance of wrinkles. They recommend facial cosmetic acupuncture for people over the age of 35. It is a minimally-invasive, non-surgical technique with few, if any, side effects.

There are acupuncture techniques that specifically target the signs of aging, such as:

- loose jowls
- double chins
- deep wrinkles
- under-eye bags
- droopy eyelids

Your acupuncturist will customize your 'rejuvenating acupuncture facial' session according to your wishes. At the end of twelve sessions (two per week), you may see a tighter jawline, taut facial skin, diminished jowls, reduced wrinkles and lifted eyelids.

Some acupuncturists give patients a homeopathic medicine to take on the evening before the treatment, to minimize the chances of bruising. The procedure takes about 30 minutes. Any bruises fade in a few days.

The patient lies down while the acupuncturist places needles in both earlobes to help reduce pain. The ears are said to be an 'anesthetic zone'. Next, needles are placed, one by one, into the cheeks, jaw, chin, temple, scalp and brows. If the body is also being treated, needles may be placed in the feet and hands.

Treatment of the scalp is the 'facelift' part of the cosmetic acupuncture process and involves lifting and pulling the skin from the jaw and then pinning it higher up on the scalp near the forehead using the needles. Although it sounds painful, it is not.

For those with deeper wrinkles, acupuncturists use a special technique involving fine intra-dermal needles to lift the skin and stimulate collagen activity.

After 20 minutes, the needles are carefully removed. Ice pads are applied, followed by a soothing antiseptic massage.

The advantage of cosmetic acupuncture is that improvement is instantly noticeable. A maintenance session about once every six months is recommended in order to retain the benefits.

FACE THERAPY:
COSMETIC TATTOOING (PERMANENT MAKEUP)

Cosmetic tattooing is also known as 'semi-permanent makeup', 'permanent makeup' or 'micro pigmentation'. It is not really permanent, because the skin of the face renews itself rapidly, and gradually loses ink over time. Results can last up to two years but they vary depending on the client's exposure to sun, and resistance to pigment. People who wish to maintain the look should have their tattoos refreshed annually.

This procedure is intended to accentuate the shape and color of facial features. It is useful for people who cannot wear standard makeup due to allergies, or who have lost their eyebrows/eyelashes due to medical treatment or some other cause; who are unable to apply makeup correctly for some reason, or who merely wish to avoid the daily routine of makeup application and removal. Topical anesthetic is applied to the skin before and sometimes during treatment, to relieve any discomfort.

Cosmetic tattooing is an art. It should be performed by a qualified cosmetic tattooist; preferably one who is experienced in makeup artistry. Choose a technician who has studied the face, its structure, its symmetry and characteristics, and who will take into account your and personality. What looks good on one face may be unflattering on another.

Facial features that can be enhanced include –

Eyebrow Tattooing

The shape and position of the eyebrows influence the overall symmetry of the face. Eyebrows frame the eyes. Their width can make the face appear wider or narrower.

An experienced cosmetic tattooist should examine the bone structure and eyebrow hair-growth pattern of each client to appropriately match their look. The proposed design should then be drawn onto the face with a fine-tipped pen, so that the client, looking into a mirror, can approve the design or request changes.

A slender tattoo needle is used to fill in the eyebrows with natural-looking hair strokes. The technician will weave new lines amongst the existing hair for a soft and subtle enhancement. If there is little to no hair then they may use a three-dimensional technique where darker and lighter pigments are used alongside one another to give a life-like appearance, as if the hair is bouncing off the skin.

Brow design, strokes, lengths, curvature, direction, arch and length of the brow play an essential part in a achieving a successful result.

Modern tattoo effects include 'feathering': Fine strokes which resemble individual hairs are tattooed into the skin. This gives a natural-looking appearance. The tattoo blends well with any natural eyebrow hairs that are still present.

Eyeliner Tattooing

Tattooed eyeliner is used by people who wish to avoid smudged and uneven eyeliners, who have eyesight problems that hinder the accurate application of makeup, or who are allergic to conventional makeup. Eyeliner tattooing is also an alternative to standard makeup for contact lens wearers. Flecks of makeup falling into one's eyes is irritating even at the best of times, but for wearers of contact lenses it can cause bigger problems by sticking to the lenses.

Permanent, tattooed eyeliner can define the eyes and suggest the look of fuller lashes. It can look as natural or as sophisticated as you want, depending on the design you select

There is a variety of colors and styles from which to choose, so that you can achieve the results you desire. Lines can be thin, medium or thick. Effects include:

- defined eyeliners
- eyeliner with shadows
- 'soft-lash' enhancements
- dramatic pigmented 'lashes'
- 'tails'
- 'wings'
- a 'smudgy' look

A kohl-like eyeliner known as 'mucosal eyeliner' can also be applied with cosmetic tattooing.

Eyelash Tattooing

Lash enhancement is a subtle method of tattooing pigment onto the skin between the eyelashes. The lashes then appear thicker, lusher and darker. This procedure is a useful alternative to eyelash extensions, which can sometimes result in loss of lashes and allergies to the glue. Effects include shadowing of color for a soft, 'natural' look, or a bold, well-defined line.

Lip Tattooing

With cosmetic tattooing, the lips can look fuller and possess youthful color without the need for constant reapplication of lipsticks and lip-liners.

* *Permanent lipliner:* A permanent lipliner tattoo can redefine lip shape, correct asymmetrical lips or add fullness.

* *Full lip color:* This is the most popular tattoo treatment for lips. Treated lips retain their enhanced shape and tint. Clients can choose their own color. A wide range of lip tattoo inks is available, varying from vivid hues to a natural shade.

* *Lip line and blend:* This technique outlines the lip shape then blends the color from the lip line onto the lips, making the outline less obvious. A 'lip line and color blend' tattoo makes it easier to apply lipstick and ensures a good lip shape all the time.

Camouflage Tattooing

Cosmetic tattooing is also used to minimize facelift scars and correct loss of skin pigmentation.

Areola Tattooing

Following reconstructive or breast cancer surgery, cosmetic tattooing can recreate the appearance of the areola and nipple.

FACE THERAPY: EAR RESHAPING

Ear pinning or ear reshaping (pinnaplasty or otoplasty) is a type of cosmetic surgery used to treat protruding ears. Ears may not be part of the face, but they can affect the way the face looks. For example, ears that stick out from the sides of the head are unlikely to have any adverse health effects; but they can be a source of embarrassment and distress.

Ear reshaping involves remodeling the ear cartilage, usually either by ear splinting (for infants) or surgical remodeling. The surgeon can create natural-looking folds and position the ears closer to the head.

FACE THERAPY: EYEBROW GROOMING

Many treatments exist for maintaining or recreating the shape and position of the eyebrows. These include plucking, waxing, threading, electrolysis, cosmetic tattooing, eyebrow transplant and dyeing.

Plucking
Plucking is one way to remove eyebrow hairs from where they are not wanted. It is usually done by simply gripping each hair with tweezers and pulling it out by the root. This process is rendered easier if you apply a warm, damp washcloth to the skin prior to plucking. The hairs will grow back; plucking is only a temporary solution.

Waxing
Waxing is another way to pull out eyebrow hairs by the roots. Warm wax is applied to the treatment area. The hairs stick to the wax as it cools and hardens. With one quick movement, the wax is stripped away, taking the hairs with it. One disadvantage of waxing is that the action of tugging in an area where skin is thinner and more delicate may cause damage. Hair will also eventually grow back after waxing.

Threading
Threading is done by tying the ends of a long piece of thread together and twisting the middle section a few times into a spiral.

When the thread is moved back and forth against the skin, the twisted part grabs the eyebrow hairs and pulls them out by the roots.

Electrolysis

If you want to shape your eyebrows other than by waxing, threading or tweezing, you might consider electrolysis. One of the advantages of electrolysis for eyebrow grooming is that the end result is permanent. After all sessions have been completed, you don't need any further treatment.

Electrolysis can be used on any skin type or color of hair, and because it targets hair follicles individually, it is very precise. Electrolysis is considered safer than permanent eyebrow hair removal by laser, which can potentially damage the eyes if used incorrectly. It also has the advantage over a laser of working well on all skin and hair colors.

Disadvantages include the facts that it can be time-consuming and costly. It can also be rather painful, and if not performed by a trained technician, can cause skin discoloration.

Cosmetic tattooing

If your eyebrows are sparse or non-existent due to medical reasons or over-plucking or aging, you may consider eyebrow tattooing.

There is a wide range of pigment colors available, and modern techniques can make tattooed eyebrows look very natural. It can be, however, quite expensive.

Choose a trained and experienced technician and make sure you agree on the shape you prefer before the treatment goes ahead. Learn more by reading "Eyebrow Tattooing" on page 118.

Tinting/Dyeing

Eyebrow tinting or dyeing is the process of coloring the eyebrow hairs using a particular shade or a variety of shades. It can be a temporary effect which is refreshed daily, or a semi-permanent effect. This treatment is an alternative to using makeup such as brow pencils, powders, or tinted brow gels for eyebrow grooming. It can be performed in beauty salons or at home.

Tinting your eyebrows can improve their appearance, making them look more defined. In turn this can enhance your facial features. It can also make the eyebrows look thicker, and cover grey hairs.

As a general rule, when choosing your eyebrow tint look for a color that is the same as your hair color except a little darker.

Temporary Eyebrow Tinting

Temporary eyebrow tinting needs to be refreshed daily. It is simply a matter of applying the color when needed, and washing it off at night before you go to bed.

Temporary eyebrow tints come in a range of colors and can be purchased as liquids or gels from your local pharmacy, drugstore or cosmetic shop, or online. They are applied using applicators, which are often sold bundled with the tints.

Semi-permanent Eyebrow Tinting

People who lack confidence in their ability to apply temporary tints, or who want an effect that lasts longer, might consider semi-permanent eyebrow tinting. The results of this remain visible for 4 to 8 weeks, before slowly fading.

Semi-permanent eyebrow tinting can be done at home; however it is recommended that you consult a professional esthetician who can help you choose the appropriate tint color.

Eyebrow Transplant

Eyebrow transplants are used when the natural eyebrow hair has become sparse or has disappeared altogether. They are a permanent replacement for cosmetic tattooing, eyebrow tinting, or drawing on your eyebrows every day.

During the eyebrow transplant procedure, the patient's own hair follicles are moved from another body area to the brow area. Once implanted in in their new location, the follicles grow completely normal, strong, healthy hairs. Generally, the follicles are taken from the back or sides of the head.

The procedure can take between 2 to 3 hours, depending on the number of grafts transplanted. The surgeon can transplant 50 to 150 or more grafts, depending on the patient's needs. The procedure is carried out under local anesthetic, combined with mild sedation and is practically painless.

Afterwards, patients may experience some mild discomfort in the areas that were treated, but analgesics can help relive these symptoms.

Immediately following the treatment, the brows and donor area will be red and slightly swollen. No bandages are required. Most patients report that some follicles start growing hair right after the procedure. Typically, more than 90% of the grafts will survive and grow healthy, permanent eyebrow hairs in their new position.

The drawback is that the transplanted hair will continue to grow long, unlike real eyebrow hairs. These new hairs will need regular trimming to keep them short.

TIPS FOR EYEBROW GROOMING
In general your eyebrows will look best if they are a shade or two darker than the hair on your head. This slight darkening will accentuate their shape and fullness without looking unnatural. If your eyebrows are very pale, consider having them tinted.

- Refrain from drawing your eyebrows onto your face with an eyebrow pencil. This will make them look too hard and harsh. Yes, you want your eyebrows to be well-defined, but a soft look is much more attractive. Instead of pencil, apply an eye shadow powder that is a shade or two darker than your hair color. This will help make your eyebrows look fuller.

- Apply a dusting of pale eye shadow powder to the area just beneath your eyebrows. This makes your eyebrows appear to lift a little and highlights their arches, thus making your eyes look more striking.

- Have your eyebrows trimmed regularly to keep them neat. Random hairs that are out of alignment can spoil the shape of your eyebrows. If your eyebrows are long and disorderly, use eyebrow scissors to snip off the excess length. Make sure you trim the hairs in the direction of growth, so that the snipped end is at an acute angle. Eyebrow scissors with curved tips usually produce the most natural-looking result. Straight-tipped scissors can leave the snipped hairs looking too blunt. Trimming is not easy to do by yourself at home, so consider visiting a salon and employing a professional esthetician.

- You can keep your well-shaped eyebrows looking tidy and neat all day by applying a clear gel mascara. Just sweep the mascara wand lightly over your eyebrows, then brush them into shape with an eyebrow brush and wipe off any surplus gel.

- If you are waxing or plucking your eyebrows, make sure you do not remove too much hair from between them. Eyebrows that are too wide apart make your facial features look out-of-kilter and somewhat asymmetrical.

EYEBROW TOOLKIT

Suggestions for your eyebrow toolkit for home use include:

- A waxing product made specifically for use on the face.

- A pair of sharp, stainless-steel tweezers for plucking. Use tweezers with straight, slanted or pointy tips; whichever you prefer.
- Clear eyebrow gel mascara to keep stray hairs in place, as well as giving your eyebrows a glossy finish.
- Soft brow pencils to define the outline of an arch (but not to draw on the eyebrows).
- Pale eyeshadow powder to highlight the area just beneath your eyebrows.
- Eyeshadow that is a couple of shades darker than your hair to accentuate your eyebrows.
- An eyebrow brush, or 'eyebrow spoolie'. This cosmetic tool resembles a mascara wand. It is the ideal instrument to manage unruly eyebrow hairs. You can also use it to comb your eyebrows into shape before trimming them. If you cannot find an eyebrow brush, you can use a disposable mascara wand.
- A sharp pair of eyebrow scissors, if you are going to trim your eyebrows at home.

FACE THERAPY: EYELASH TREATMENTS

Eyelashes can be enhanced with:
- Cosmetic tattooing
- Devices to curl the eyelashes
- Dyes and tints to change their color (note— this is dangerous!)
- Eyelash conditioners
- Eyelash extensions to lengthen them
- Eyelash transplants
- Mascara to add length and volume and color
- Prescription drugs such as 'Latisse®'
- Prosthetics (false eyelashes), including full- and half-lashes

* Eyelash cosmetic tattooing

Learn more in the section on 'lash enhancement' under 'Cosmetic Tattooing' (page 120).

* Eyelash curling devices
An eyelash curler is a hand-operated mechanical device, sometimes called 'eyelash curling tongs', used to curl the upper eyelashes (and rarely, the lower lashes).

The device works the same way as other hair curling devices; by heating the lashes while bending them into their new shape. Some eyelash curlers are battery operated, while others must be heated by the hot air from a hair dryer.

Aficionados of eyelash curling say that the curls (which curve away from the eye, not towards it) make the eyes appear bigger and brighter and the lashes appear longer. Skillfully applied, the curling effect can alter the appearance of the eye's shape. For example, if curls are made more pronounced at the eye's outer corners, they make the eye look attractively 'upswept' - a shape that is called 'almond' or 'elvish'.

Eyelash curling devices can be used at home and require no training. Users of these devices should be careful, however. Too much tugging on the lashes while curling them can lead to eyelash shedding, and if the user accidentally pinches the eyelid they can cause injury. The heat in the device can also burn the lids and lashes.

* Eyelash dyes and tints
Eyelash dyes are dangerous. They can cause blindness. We recommend that you never use them, either at home or in a salon. They can also cause swelling, eye infections and inflammation of the eye.

Mascara has many advantages over eyelash dyes - it can not only darken them, it can also make them longer, thicker and curlier.

* Eyelash conditioners
These commercial products are formulated to increase the health, fullness and length of the lashes. Ingredients can include seed extracts,

minerals and even 'growth serums'. Beware of eye irritation, and if you purchase an eyelash conditioner, choose cruelty-free.

* Eyelash extensions

Eyelash extensions, also known as semi-permanent lashes, are artificial lashes which are professionally glued, one by one, to each of your natural eyelashes.

When applied correctly, neither the extension lash nor the glue touches the actual eyelid. The special glue is intended to hold firmly until your eyelashes naturally fall out; however it can be weakened by frequent eye-rubbing or the application of oil-based eye makeup remover.

Eyelash extensions generally remain in place for about 3-4 weeks, which is the duration of your lashes' normal growth and shedding cycle.

People use eyelash extensions to enhance the look of the eyes in the same way as mascara, but without having to apply mascara daily and remove it at night.

The artificial lashes are available in a range of lengths, colors and thicknesses. Attaching them can take up to two hours, and is should be done by a trained esthetician.

* Eyelash transplants

Eyelash transplants are just like other surgical hair transplants, such as augmentation of hair on the head by grafting hair from another part of the body.

However, since the new 'eyelashes' are hairs transplanted from the head, they will continue to grow exactly like head hair, instead of stopping at eyelash length. Therefore they will need to be trimmed regularly.

* Mascara

This is a cosmetic product which users smear along the length of their eyelashes, using a mascara 'wand'. Its purpose is to enhance the look of the eyelashes by darkening, thickening, lengthening, and/

or defining the eyelashes. Most mascara formulations are based on pigments, oils, waxes, and preservatives.

* Prescription drugs
Latisse® is a topical solution that is available on prescription. When applied to the lids, it can make the lashes grow darker, longer and fuller.

The disadvantages of Latisse® include side effects such as:
- Redness, itchiness and irritation, which disappear when you discontinue use of the drug
- Purplish-brown discoloration and pigmentation of the upper and lower eyelids
- If your eyes are hazel or blue in color, the use of Latisse can, in rare cases, permanently change their color to brown.

* False eyelashes
Also called 'temporary false eyelashes', these are designed to be worn for a short period, such as during a party or a night out. They are not meant to be worn when you are showering, sleeping or swimming.

These prosthetics, which are designed to resemble human eyelashes, adhere to the upper eyelids just above the upper lash line, or to the lower eyelids just below the lower lash line. They are stuck on with a special eyelash glue which enables them to be removed before bedtime. They can be purchased at pharmacies, drug-stores, cosmetics stores and online.

FACE THERAPY: EYE COLOR

While we are on the topic of eye appearance, it is perhaps worth noting that even the color of the eyes themselves can be enhanced or altered non-surgically, by the use of colored contact lenses.

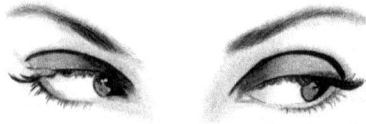

FACE THERAPY: FACELIFT SURGERY

The most noticeable signs of facial aging are the changes in position of the deep anatomical structures, including the platysma muscle, cheek fat and the orbicularis oculi muscle.

The platysma muscle is a broad expanse of muscle running from the chest and shoulder muscles, over the collarbone and upward at an angle along the sides of the neck.

The orbicularis oculi muscle is a ringlike band of muscle that surrounds the eye. Its function is to open and close the eyelids.

When these three structures age, the following signs of aging occur:

- 'Jowls' appear when the once cleanly-sculpted jawline is broken or blurred by the drooping of the platysma muscle.

- The groove running from the outer edges of the nose to the outer corners of the mouth (the nasolabial fold) becomes deeper when the cheek fat descends.

- Baggy pouches appear beneath the eyes when the orbicularis oculi muscle loses tone.

- The condition of the skin is a fourth noticeable sign of facial aging.

The acronym 'SMAS' os often used when discussing facelift surgery. This refers to the 'sub-muscular aponeurotic system'—a layer of strong, connective tissue that covers and is attached to the deeper anatomy of the face, cheeks and neck, including the platysma.

Some areas of the face, such as the nasolabial folds or marionette lines, may be better improved with wrinkle relaxants, dermal fillers, PRP injections or liposculpture. Estheticians suggest that the ideal age for a face lift is before the age of fifty.

TYPES OF FACELIFT SURGERY

Many different procedures of facelift (rhytidectomy) exist. The variations lie mostly in the type of incision, the invasiveness and the area of the face that is treated. Cosmetic surgeons endeavor to choose the right procedure or combination of procedures for each individual patient.

Traditional 'skin only' facelift

With this method only the skin of the face is lifted and not the underlying SMAS, muscles or other structures. The skin itself lacks the elasticity and laxity in older patients, which is why the results of this facelift are fairly short-lived. Usually the lift re-sags within 6 to 12 months after the procedure. The reason people consider this option is that it has fewer complications and isn't as technically demanding as the SMAS or other types of lifts.

The surgeon makes an incision in front of the ear, continuing up into the hairline. The incision curves around the bottom of the ear and then behind it, usually ending near the hairline on the back of the neck. After the incision is made, the skin is separated from the deeper tissues with a scalpel or scissors (also called undermining) over the cheeks and neck. The skin is then re-draped, and the surgeon removes an amount of excess skin (which is determined by his or her judgment and experience), before closing the skin incisions with sutures and staples.

The traditional facelift lifts and tightens only the superficial epidermal and dermal layers of the skin. It does not alter the position of the underlying fat and lax SMAS-platysma layer. It may also produce an unnatural 'stretched' look.

Surgeons sometimes remove excess underlying tissues and use deep sutures to gather up the fat and SMAS layers in small folds before stretching the skin over the top; however in the long term this does not seem to add much improvement to the results of a traditional 'skin only' facelift.

SMAS facelift
The structural SMAS layer of the facial tissues holds the cheek fat in its normal position. Surgically resuspending and securing the SMAS layer can make the face look rejuvenated, by counteracting the laxity caused by aging.

The surgeon uses 'undermining' to free the tissue layers including the SMAS layer. Then all layers are lifted upward. Excess fat is cut away or removed using liposuction. The tension placed on the SMAS layer lifts the lax neck fat and places the top skin layer in a better, more youthful-looking position. Because the lifting of the tissues happens at a deeper, supporting level, the SMAS facelift produces a close-fitting, enduring lift of the chin and jawline that does not have a 'stretched' look.

Modifications to the SMAS facelift technique have led to the development of the 'Bidirectional Facelift', the 'Composite Facelift' and 'Deep Plane Facelift.'

Bidirectional facelift

This technique, used in conjunction with the SMAS facelift method, can improve the look of the deep fold lines on the side of the nose and mouth (the naso-labial folds), and lift the mid-cheek fat pad (the malar fat pad). 'Wide superficial undermining of the upper and mid-cheek skin which is pulled laterally for correction of the nasolabial fold achieves a bidirectional facelift.'[34]

Deep-plane facelift

The SMAS lift is an effective procedure to reposition the platysma muscle; however the nasolabial fold is (according to some surgeons) better addressed by a deep plane facelift or composite facelift. The deep plane facelift differs from the SMAS lift in that it frees cheek fat and some muscles from their anchoring bone structure.

This technique has a higher risk of damaging the facial nerve.

Composite facelift

Similar to the deep plane facelift, the composite facelift involves a deeper layer of tissue being released and repositioned. The difference between these techniques is the extra repositioning and securing of the orbicularis oculi muscle (muscle around the eyes) in the composite facelift procedure.

The 'malar crescent' is a crescent-shaped bagginess that, in older faces, lies under the eye and along the upper part of the cheek. Composite facelifts can also improve the appearance of these bags.

Mid-facelift

The mid face area – the area between the cheeks – flattens as women age and makes the face look slightly more masculine. The

---

34   *Clin Plast Surg. 1983 Jul;10(3):429-40. SMAS-platysma facelift. A bidi-rectional cervicofacial rhytidectomy. Owsley JQ Jr. PMID: 6627837*

mid-face lift is recommended for people with this flattened look, who have no significant degree of jowling or sagging of the neck. In these cases, a mid-face-lift is sufficient to rejuvenate the face, as opposed to a full facelift.

The ideal candidates for a mid face-lift is when a person is in her or his forties, or if the cheeks appear to be drooping and the lip-to nose (nasolabial) area is sagging.

The surgeon makes several small incisions along the hairline and inside the mouth. This way the fatty tissue layers can be lifted and repositioned, with barely visible scars.

The fatty layer that lies over the cheekbones is also lifted and repositioned. This improves the nose-to-mouth lines and the roundness over the cheekbones.

The recovery time is comparatively short, and this procedure is often combined with a blepharoplasty (eyelid surgery).

Mini-facelift

The mini-facelift is the least invasive type of facelift. It is similar to a full facelift–the only difference is the omission of the neck lift in the mini lift procedure. It is also called the 'S' lift (because of the shape of the incision that is used), or the 'short-scar' facelift.

This lift is a more temporary solution to the aging of the face. It also entails less downtime. It is suitable for people who have deep nasolabial folds and sagging facial structures, yet who still have a firm and well-contoured neck. It is an alternative to the full facelift for people with premature aging.

The surgeon usually makes an incision from the hairline around the ear, so that scars will be hidden in the natural fold of the skin.

The mini lift can be performed with an endoscope[35]. The surgeon repositions the soft tissues, then sutures the skin with small stitches to hold it in place.

Ribbon lift

Ribbon lifting (not to be confused with thread lifting) is a facelift procedure during which absorbable 'ribbon' implants are inserted beneath the skin of the face, neck and/or scalp.

Ribbon implants look like a piece of translucent plastic with spikes jutting from one side. They are manufactured in varying shapes and sizes depending on their particular purpose. Not all of them look like ribbons, though we are classifying them all under 'ribbon lifting' due to the fact that they are all made from the same material. Some if these implants are triangular in shape, some resemble a small dog-collar, and others look like miniature, tined platforms no bigger than a fingernail.

During ribbon lifting treatment the surgeon makes a small incision, through which he or she lifts and repositions the skin. The ribbon implant is then inserted, and the spikes are fixed into the platysma muscle to hold the skin in its new position. Trade names of ribbon lifting include Endotine®.

Ribbon lifts can be used in the following ways:

Ribbon Lifting Endoscopic Brow Lift

The patient is put under intravenous sedation or general anesthesia. The procedure generally takes between one and two hours and is usually performed in the surgeon's clinic.

---

35   An endoscope is a medical device consisting of a long, thin tube which can be threaded inside the patient's body. A light and sometimes a tiny camera are attached. Endoscopes are used to look inside a body cavity or organ.

A tiny camera (on an endoscope) is inserted into one of several tiny incisions placed just behind the hairline, giving the surgeon a view of the muscles and tissues beneath the skin.

The surgeon then inserts another instrument through another of the incisions to lift and reposition the skin. A ribbon implant is used to securely hold the tissue in place during the healing process. Typical 'downtime' is a week or two.

Ribbon Lifting Open Brow Lift

This is a more conventional surgical technique. Again, the patient is put under intravenous sedation or general anesthesia. The procedure generally takes between one and two hours and is usually performed in the surgeon's clinic.

The surgeon makes an incision behind the hairline and above the ears and continues toward the top of the head. He or she pulls the skin of the brow and forehead into place, and may also cut off any excess skin and muscle that causes wrinkling.

A triangular implant is used to securely hold the tissue in place during the healing process.

Combination Brow Lift

A combination of endoscopic and open surgical techniques may be used.

Ribbon Lifting Direct Brow Lift

For this procedure, patients are usually given local anesthesia with conscious sedation. Treatment takes about 30 minutes. It is usually combined with conventional blepharoplasty (cosmetic eyelid surgery).

First, the surgeon makes an incision in the crease of the upper eyelid and removes excess fat, skin and sometimes muscle. This completes the blepharoplasty.

Using the same incision used for the blepharoplasty, the surgeon releases the soft tissues under the brow and forehead. He or she then affixes a small implant called a 'transbleph device' to the bone near the eyebrow, to hold the brow and underlying tissues in their new position until healing is complete, after which the implant is absorbed naturally by the body.

Ribbon Lifting Mid-face Lift

During a mid-face lift, the surgeon inserts an endoscope through a tiny incision. He or she uses a surgical instrument to lift the underlying tissues. The ribbon implant is then inserted beneath the soft tissue to hold the cheek's soft tissue in place.

Mid-face lift surgery is usually performed in office-based surgical suites. The patient can receive either general anesthesia or local anesthesia and sedation, and can usually return home on the same day.

Ribbon Lifting Lower Face/Neck Lift

The surgeon makes a small incision in the hairline or behind the ear. Through this incision, the surgeon creates a space, like a tunnel, between the skin and deeper tissues. The ribbon's spikes are then placed in the deeper tissue, permitting the surgeon to pull the underlying tissues into a new position.

The surgeon then sutures (stitches) the opposite end of the ribbon to strong underlying tissue, to anchor it in place. He or she cuts off any excess skin and closes the incision.

Subperiosteal facelift

The word 'periosteum' refers to a membrane that covers the outer surface of nearly all of our bones, and to which our muscles are attached. The subperiosteal face lift, a procedure designed to rejuvenate the upper and middle thirds of the face, is done by vertically lifting the soft tissues of the face, completely separating them from the underlying facial bones and elevating them to a more esthetically pleasing position. This technique can improve the appearance of deep nasolabial folds and sagging cheeks. It is often combined with standard facelift techniques. Results are long-lasting and suitable for all adult age groups.

One difference between this and other facelifts is that patients will usually experience a longer period of facial swelling after the procedure.

MACS facelift
The term MACS-lift–or Minimal Access Cranial Suspension lift–allows for the correction of drooping facial tissues through a short, small incision. The surgeon is able to elevate the facial tissues vertically, by suspending them from above.

Overall, the MACS-lift surgery is safer than many other kinds of facelifts because less skin is raised. This means that there is less risk of bleeding and nerve damage.

The operation also takes less time, lasting around 2.5 hours instead of the 3.5 hours that most other facelifts require.

There is also a shorter recovery period, 2–3 weeks instead of 3–4 weeks. Finally, the outcome of the MACS-lift is very natural-looking while the traditional facelift often results in a stretched, 'windswept' look.[36]

Brow Lift
A forehead lift, also sometimes referred to as a brow lift, is a surgical procedure to change the position of the soft tissues of the forehead. It is used to rejuvenate the appearance of the upper face and reduce sagging of skin around the eyebrows and above the nose. Multiple surgical approaches and methods have been developed for brow lifts, and more than one may be used in combination by surgeons wishing to elevate the forehead skin.

For more information, visit our section on Brow Lifting (page 112).

---

36   *Rhytidectomy - Wikipedia, the free encyclopedia. Article retrieved November 2014.*

ⓘ Chin Reshaping Surgery

Chin reshaping is used to improve the appearance of a jaw that might be considered over-large or over-small or asymmetrical.

Sometimes the jaws may need adjustment with a combination of braces and jaw surgery. This technique is known as orthognathic surgery.

Large chins can be surgically pared back, while small chins can be augmented with artificial chin implants, or by means of genioplasty. With genioplasty, the surgeon makes cut in the bone, moves the bone forward and wires it in place. The bones eventually heal into the new position and the remodeled chin becomes a normal component of the facial bones.

There are, of course, risks and complications with any kind of surgery. Your doctor will advise you on this subject.

POTENTIAL COMPLICATIONS OF FACELIFT SURGERY

The most common complication of facial surgery can be bleeding, which usually requires a return to the operating room. Less common but potentially serious complications may include damage to the facial nerves, necrosis of the skin flaps, infection or an adverse reaction to the anesthetic.

Hematoma is the most commonly seen complication after facelift surgery. Arterial bleeding can cause the most dangerous hematomas, as this type can lead to dyspnea (shortness of breath). If a hematoma is going to occur, it will almost always do so within the first 24 hours after the facelift surgery.

Nerve injury can be temporary or permanent. Harm can be done to either the sensory or the motor nerves of the face.

Necrosis, the premature death of cells in living tissue, can occur after a facelift operation. Smoking increases the risk of skin necrosis 12-fold.

Scarring is considered a complication of facelift surgery. Hypertrophic scars can appear.

A facelift requires skin incisions; however, the incisions in front of and behind the ear are usually inconspicuous. Hair loss in the portions of the incision within the hair-bearing scalp can occur after a facelift. Distortion of the hairline can result. Men can lose facial hair after a facelift procedure. In men, the sideburns can be pulled backwards and upwards, resulting in an unnatural appearance if appropriate techniques are not employed to address this issue. Achieving a natural appearance following surgery in men can be more challenging due to their hair-bearing skin.

In both men and women, one of the signs of having had a facelift can be an earlobe which is pulled forwards and/or distorted. Also, if the surgeon is not skilled, the patient's face can assume a pulled-back, 'windswept' appearance. This appearance can also be due to some changes in bone structure due to aging.

The vector forces at work in a facelift will lower the ears as well as change the angle of the ears. Ears may be lowered as much as 1 cm (0.4 inches) and the change in the angle can be as much as 10 degrees.[37]

FACE THERAPY: MINIMALLY-INVASIVE 'FACELIFTS'

THREAD LIFT

The 'thread lift' may also be known as 'barbed suture lift', 'contour thread lift' or 'feather lift'. Thread lifting is a minimally invasive surgical procedure, which is often used for people who seek minor improvements to sagging or laxity in the areas of the eyes, midface, jowls, forehead, neck and nasolabial fold.

---

37   *Ibid.*

Thread lifting cannot, of course, replicate the dramatic results of surgical facelifts. Threads (sutures) only provide some lift. However, when combined with other treatments such as erbium laser resurfacing, fat transfer to refill the hollowed aged cheeks and dark under-eye circles, or liposuction to remove a heavy neck, jowls or double chin, a thread lift may provide satisfactory cosmetic results.

Since the invention of the first short, barbed thread lift sutures in the late 1990s, different techniques have appeared on the market. These include 'Woffles lifting', which uses long thread; APTOS® and WAPTOS® suture lifting, Isse unidirectional barbed-threads lifting, and Silhouette Lift®.

The procedure
The threads are inserted and positioned while the patient is under local anesthesia. Using a hollow guiding needle, the surgeon guides barbed threads into the deep tissue of the face. After removal of the needle, the thread remains in position and attaches itself to the subcutaneous tissue. The surgeon then pulls this same tissue into the desired position and secures it there. The ends of the thread are drawn and trimmed short. They disappear under the skin.

No skin is cut away. The threads and the barbs (cogs) along them are what keep the lift in place. The barbs on one end of the thread anchor themselves to the underlying skin tissues and the barbs on the other end grab and gently lift the skin in the desired direction. Thus, the facial tissue and skin is gathered into place. The lift heals into position after several days, through the natural connective tissue.

Suitable candidates
Thread lifting is generally suitable for those who:
- —do not have significant amounts of loose skin. This usually means patients below the age of 45 or 50.
- —do not have very thin skin. In thin-skinned patients the suture may be visible.

- • — are not overweight or very thin.
- • — are in good health and not taking any medication that thins the blood.

A good way to check whether you are suitable is to gently lift and push back the skin of your mid-face towards the ears, using your fingers. The amount of skin bunching you get indicates the amount you will get post-procedure. Too much means you are not a good candidate.

Potential risks and complications

Specific complications of thread lifting include puckering skin, the visibility of the threads beneath the skin and the appearance of lumps. Also there is the problem of skin bunching around the ears, where the loose skin is pulled to. Treatments to address these effects range from oral medications, to using clear threads, to surgical intervention.

Duration of results

The duration of the result varies, depending on the age of the patient at the time of the procedure, the type of threads used, the degree of skin sagging, and the number of threads used. Some practitioners claim that it can last from 3 to 5 years, after which time the positive effect is gradually lost.

Researchers have been less than enthusiastic about the results of thread lifts. A 2009 study by R.F. Abraham concluded, 'The thread-lift provides only limited short-term improvement that may be largely attributed to post-procedural edema (swelling) and inflammation. Our results objectively demonstrate the poor long-term sustainability of the thread-lift procedure. Given these findings, as well as the measurable risk of adverse events and patient discomfort, we cannot justify further use of this procedure for facial rejuvenation.'[38]

In 2010 medical researcher J.D. Rachel concluded, 'The goal for new procedures should be to deliver predictable long-term results while providing less morbidity, less downtime, and greater patient satisfaction. The results of this study indicate that the barbed suture lift was unable to accomplish these goals.[39]

Thread Types
There are three main types of threads used for lifts:
* Permanent non-absorbable barbed threads
* Removable non-absorbable threads
* Absorbable threads

Permanent non-absorbable barbed threads.
This type of thread will not be reabsorbed into the body or dissolved over time. They remain in place. The thread material consists of non-absorbable monofilament sutures which are biocompatible but permanent.

Permanent, non-absorbable threads are used to:

* Lift and support the droopy areas of the brow
* Lift and support lax areas of the face
* Lift and support the sagging areas of the neck
* Lift sagging eyebrows
* Adjust asymmetric eyebrows
* Reposition and support sagging cheeks

---

38   *Arch Facial Plast Surg. 2009 May-Jun;11(3):178-83. doi: 10.1001/ archfacial. 2009.10. Thread-lift for facial rejuvenation: assessment of long-term results. Abraham RF, DeFatta RJ, Williams EF 3rd.*

39   *Dermatol Surg. 2010 Mar;36(3):348-54. doi: 10.1111/j.1524-4725.2009.01442.x. Epub 2010 Jan 19.*
Incidence of complications and early recurrence in 29 patients after facial rejuvenation with barbed suture lifting.
Rachel JD1, Lack EB, Larson B.

- Lift drooping soft tissue of the mid and lower face
- Smooth out premature skin aging
- Lift and support early 'jowling'

The surgeon anchors threads in the hairline via an incision in the temple area. The threads are inserted in precise locations using a long needle, and once inserted under the skin, they open in an umbrella like fashion to form a support structure that gently lifts and repositions the tissues into a more vertical and youthful position.

After the lift effect has been secured, the surgeon removes the needle. The end of the thread is cut and knotted, allowing it to retract deep beneath the skin where it cannot be felt or seen. The non-absorbable threads stay within the deep tissues and provide support.

The procedure usually takes less than 30 to 60 minutes to complete, depending on the number of threads used. Patients are able to go home soon after the procedure.

Permanent non-absorbable thread lifting is a stand-alone procedure. However, it is not uncommon to combine it with other techniques including dermal fillers to enhance volume, muscle relaxing injections of botulinum toxin, or chemical peels, microdermabrasion and laser and light therapy to improve skin texture.

After the procedure, most patients experience a small amount of bruising or swelling for 1—7 days. Most patients can return to normal activities the next day, using makeup as a concealer. Pain and discomfort are said to be minimal with this technique and most patients need take only take over-the-counter medication for pain relief. In most cases, ice compresses are recommended for the first 24—48 hours.

When performed by a qualified, experienced physician, the procedure is very safe. Problems are uncommon and usually easily correctable. Since a thread lift is performed under local anesthesia, there are none of the risks associated with general anesthesia.

One potential adverse outcome is that sometimes threads can be seen beneath the skin.

Results will vary depending on the extent of sagging and the degree of lifting desired, as well as the technique of the physician and the number of threads used in each area treated. Some patients may require more than one treatment session to achieve a noticeable improvement.

The duration of the effect varies, depending on the age of the patient at the time of the procedure, the degree of sagging, and the number of threads used. Permanent non-absorbable thread lifting generally lasts 3-5 years and can be repeated.

Trade names include 'APTOS® Lift' (anti-ptosis) and 'Silhouette® Lift'.

Removable non-absorbable threads

Strands of 'prolene' monofilament thread, with tiny notches cut into their sides, are threaded into the deep skin layers under the drooping facial skin. These threads are anchored under secure points in the tissues of the fronto-occipitalis muscle (which covers part of the skull) and the temporalis muscles (broad, fan-shaped muscle on each side of the head, above the ears). Dropped facial skin is then elevated onto the barbed threads, where it stays elevated because of the barbs. There is no removal of skin.

If a patient is dissatisfied with the results, removable non-absorbable prolene threads can be removed, after which the patient's face returns to its position prior to treatment.

Effects can last for a number of years, after which the improvement is gradually lost.

Trade names include 'Contour Lift'®.

Absorbable threads

Absorbable threads have a high bio-tolerance. They slowly dissolve over a period of 12—15 months. Absorbable thread lifting works in two ways.

- It immediately lifts sagging tissue via the action of the threads, which become fixed by the skins natural fibrosis.
- As it dissolves, it regenerates and volumizes the face. The process of thread breakdown stimulates the skin's natural

production of collagen and hyaluronic acid. Consequently, the skin becomes more moisturized, elastic, smooth and firm. This effect can remain visible for as long as 5—6 years.

Absorbable thread lifting suits patients aged 30—60 who wish to rejuvenate their face and neck. The threads can lift drooping skin in the brow, cheek, mid face, jawline/jowls, chin and neck area, and even the nose.

The procedure usually takes 15—40 minutes and is performed in the surgeon's office. Local anesthesia is used only at the entry and exit points of the thread, and a surgical incision is not necessary.

After treatment some needle marks will show up on the face and there may be some 'bunching' of the skin which will resolve in a few days. Most patients are able to hide any bruises or needle marks with makeup, and they can return to normal activities the following day.

Because absorbable threads are not anchored, they cannot give as dramatic an instant lift as with the non-absorbable threads. However if used in combination with dermal fillers, wrinkle relaxing inject-ables and skin tightening treatments (e.g. laser Fraxel, Thermage) this treatment can give impressive results.

According to studies, skin improvement continues for five months after treatment and lasts up to two years.

Trade names of the absorbable thread technique include 'Happy Lift'® and 'Silhouette Soft'®.

FACE THERAPY: NON-SURGICAL 'FACELIFTS'

Many people want a facelift, but feel reluctant to undergo invasive surgical procedures. They wish to enjoy the benefits of looking younger, but would rather avoid hospitalization and anesthesia, not to mention a prolonged recovery period away from their social lives until the healing is complete.

The good news is that surgery is not the only option. Non-surgical facelifts can be very effective for rejuvenation and face-shaping. Relatively quick treatments, sometimes called 'lunch time lifts' can give you a more youthful, refreshed look without surgery, general anesthetic or prolonged recovery time.

The results of non-surgical facelifts do not last as long as surgical procedures, nor can they replicate them, although they can come close. They do not 'lift' the face the in the same way. Instead, they smooth and tighten the skin, replace volume and reduce wrinkles.

Non-surgical cosmetic treatments for the face include:

- Injectables such as dermal fillers, muscle relaxers (eg. Botox) and 'liquid face lifts'
- Skin surface treatments, including chemical peels and microdermabrasion
- Laser, intense pulsed light (IPL) and other heat treatments.

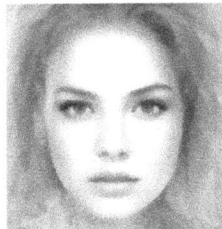

NON-SURGICAL 'FACELIFTS' – TECHNIQUES THAT WORK

As we age our faces acquire expression lines, lose fat volume and bone structure, lose elasticity, begin to sag, and suffer from sun damage. There is no single treatment that addresses all these issues and works for everyone, so a cosmetic physician might suggest that you have more than one. You could, for instance, choose from:

Minimally invasive techniques

- Wrinkle/muscle relaxers to treat forehead wrinkles, crow's feet, jawline and sagging eyebrows. See page 183.
- Dermal fillers for marionettes (indentations on each side of the lips, which can make you look sad). See page 162.
- Dermal fillers for nasolabial folds (those deep grooves that run from the nose to the mouth). See page 162.
- Dermal fillers to replace volume in the lips and cheeks.

Non-surgical techniques. (See also ""Part 4: Skin Therapy" on page 184.)

- Laser, plasma or vacuum treatments to increase facial collagen and elasticity.
- Laser treatments, photodynamic therapy, chemical peels and topical creams to reduce skin discoloration.
- Infrared light therapy, chemical peels or IPL or to erase fine lines and improve skin texture.
- Ultrasound therapy to tighten sagging muscles.
- Laser liposuction (non-invasive) techniques that break down fat deposits around the jawline, giving a cleaner, more sculpted look.
- Microcurrent therapy to treat wrinkles and sagging skin.
- Laser therapy to remove skin tags.
- Microdermabrasion for skin resurfacing and scar removal.

Ⓘ FACE THERAPY: FACIAL FAT TRANSFER

Fat transfer, also called 'fat grafting', involves harvesting fat from one part of the body and inserting it into another. Advantages of using your own fat to increase volume are:

- There is no chance of allergic reaction to your own tissues.
- It looks and feels natural.
- It is cheaper than using large volumes of synthetic material.
- Fat can be safely stored frozen and later re-injected for further fat transfer treatments.
- Stem cells found in fat rejuvenate the skin, making it thicker, smoother and brighter–like young skin.

A wide range of people may benefit from fat transfer. As we age, our facial fat shifts and sometimes decreases. Facial skin sags and deflates, partly because of a reduction in fat holding it out and up.

People who wish to minimize the signs of advancing years may dislike like the hollow, deflated appearance of the cheeks and the tissues around the mouth. The lost volume can be replaced with fat from another part of the body. An added advantage is the removal of material from an area of the body that may be too fat.

Fat transfer works very well to treat loss of volume in the face, but fine lines and wrinkles are best treated with dermal fillers.

Facial fat transfer can address the following issues:

- Gaunt cheeks.
- Hollows under the eye.
- Hollows at the temple.
- Lack of volume along the jawline.

ADVANTAGES OF FAT TRANSFER OVER DERMAL FILLERS

Dermal fillers are thicker and more viscous than fat, so when they are used to add volume to sagging faces they look natural when that face is expressionless, but may look unnaturally plump and immobile, or 'overstuffed' when the person talks or laughs.

Another advantage of fat over dermal fillers is that fillers generally only last for a maximum of twelve months but fat can last much longer.

THE FAT TRANSFER PROCEDURE

The patient is given sedation and local anesthetic. The area to be harvested is then injected with a special solution that makes the fat easier to remove.

The surgeon makes a 2mm incision in the fat-harvesting area then inserts a cannula with which to remove the fat. The harvested fat is concentrated before being injected into the treatment areas.

The procedure usually takes around an hour and patients can go home soon afterwards.

Generally, recovery time is relatively short. Most patients have swelling in the area (especially the face) for 2 or 3 days, but can usually return to work after 5 to 7 days. No special dressings or sutures are necessary. The doctor may prescribe antibiotics to reduce the chances of infection. Pain is usually minimal and controlled with over-the-counter pain medication.

With early facial fat transfer techniques, most of the fat injected—up to 70 per cent—disappeared pretty rapidly, being absorbed into the body. Recently, however, improvements in the technique mean nearly all the fat injected into the face survives.

Transferred fat survives when it gains a blood supply in its new location. This gives it a source of oxygen and nutrients, which permits it to continue existing indefinitely. If the transferred fat does not receive a blood supply in the first few weeks after surgery, the body will slowly break it down and absorb it. Thus the cosmetic improvements will disappear.

Successful fat transfer surgery needs to be done with skill and precision, to make sure that the fat which is harvested is not damaged by the harvesting process, and that the fat is re-injected in a way that maximizes the potential for blood vessels to grow into it (neovascularization).

It is to be expected that even when neovascularization occurs, it may not affect all the transferred fat, some of which will naturally be absorbed by the body. The amount that remains varies between individual patients, but generally about half of the injected fat remains for longer than three months. After that time has elapsed, the remaining volume of fat may last for years.

If more volume enhancement is required then any harvested fat that has been stored can be used.

Because the amount of fat retained by the body varies, some people need two or three treatment sessions to achieve the effect they want.

Side effects may occur, such as scarring. For most people the scars from the removal process heal very well. As the body's natural healing processes remodel the tissues, they virtually disappear after a few months. The tiny injection site wounds heal after about a week.

Not all patients are suitable for a fat transfer procedure, and you should consult with your doctor to assess your suitability, based on your medical history and general health and fitness. A consultation will also allow you to discuss the risks and complications that can accompany any surgical or invasive procedure. It is suggested that before proceeding, you should seek a second medical opinion.

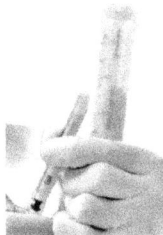

FACE THERAPY: FACIAL SKIN TIGHTENING

Skin has to be extremely elastic, because it must stretch as we move, change facial expressions, and grow. In the case of weight loss, skin has to shrink. Skin, however, is not like a rubber suit covering the entire body. It is an organ and, just like all the other organs in your body, it is composed of cells.

Different layers of skin have different types of cells. Although the cells on the outer part (the epidermis) are constantly being lost and replaced with new cells, the cells beneath the epidermis are more permanent.

These layers of the skin, called the dermis and subdermis or hypodermis, are made up of elastic connective tissues, fibers, blood vessels and various components that can stretch or contract depending on how they are treated.

When you lose weight, and especially when you lose weight very quickly, these elastic components of skin not only lose the layers of fat that keep them stretched out over your body, but they may also lack enough time for their elasticity to adapt to your new shape.

In addition to weight loss, other factors such as increasing age, poor nutrition, pregnancy, dehydration, excessive sun exposure, air pollution and smoking can all affect elasticity and give you that baggy-skin appearance.

SURGICAL SKIN TIGHTENING

The skin of the face can be made to appear tighter by means of facelift surgery. Surgery involves separating the skin from the underlying tissues, pulling it back and up, repositioning it and cutting off any excess.

This procedure makes the skin appear to be tighter, despite the fact that there has been no increase of collagen in the tissue.

Learn more in our section on facelift surgery (page 130).

ℛMINIMALLY INVASIVE SKIN TIGHTENING
Microneedling Radiofrequency Skin Tightening

Microneedling radiofrequency technology is minimally-invasive, and is what is termed a 'walk-in, walk-out' procedure. It is commonly used to tighten loose or sagging skin on the abdomen, under the arms, under the eyes, and on the cheeks, mid-face, jaw line, and neck.

During the procedure your clinician rolls a hand-held device across your skin. The device uses multiple needles less than 0.25mm in diameter, to pierce the skin and create tiny injuries deep below the surface. This causes a heating action that immediately tightens skin tissues and structures. These dermal injuries lead to new collagen formation via the body's normal skin repair mechanisms.

Microneedling radiofrequency facial skin tightening also perforates and softens fibrous scar tissue, enabling the formation of new collagen. The new collagen fills sunken scars and wrinkles from the bottom up, lifting the depressions so that they become level with the surrounding skin.

Over time, the skin produces new and remodeled collagen. This further tightens the tissues, resulting in smoother skin and a more youthful appearance. This process takes 2—3 months to produce visible results. It can also help thicken thin, crêpey skin.

Results vary depending on age and skin condition. The number of treatments required varies with each individual. Some people require only a few treatments, while others require more treatments at four-week intervals.

While pain tolerance varies from person to person, most people have little pain with microneedling radiofrequency treatment. Numbing cream can also be used to help reduce discomfort. The procedure is not accompanied by any significant side effects, though the patient's skin will be red for 1—3 days. Patients can resume regular activities immediately after treatment, with no downtime or special follow-up care.

Some brand names of microneedling radiofrequency skin tightening include: Derma Roller®, Dermapen®, INTRAcel® and Fractional RF Microneedle (FRM).

NON-SURGICAL SKIN TIGHTENING
Radiofrequency Skin Tightening

Radiofrequency facial skin tightening (also called 'thermal skin tightening') delivers fuller, plumper skin with no 'downtime'. It is suitable for anyone who would like to firm their skin and refine the appearance of fine lines and wrinkles. It can also be used as a preventative treatment for skin that is starting to show the signs of aging.

Radiofrequency skin tightening has three main effects on the skin:
- Tissue retraction: The generated heat immediately tightens the skin.
- New collagen formation: By the heating of the dermis, new collagen production is stimulated.
- Improved circulation: Radiofrequency skin tightening improves blood and lymphatic flow.

This treatment is said to be a relaxing and pleasurable experience. It involves a radiofrequency device gently heating the skin to about 41 degrees Celsius. At this temperature, the collagen fibers in the skin shrink, leading to tightening of the skin.

After a radiofrequency facial skin tightening session, the redness and heat in the treated skin disappear within 30 minutes.

A course of 10 weekly treatments is recommended. After that, maintenance treatments should be undertaken every twelve weeks.

Some names of radiofrequency facial skin tightening treatments include: CPT (Comfort Pulse Technology™) Thermage®, Pelleve Skin Tightening®, Thermal Skin Tightening, Venus Freeze® and Bodytite®.

Carbon Dioxide (CO2) Laser Resurfacing

Carbon dioxide lasers are used to tighten skin and also to resurface skin for the reduction of wrinkles, sun damage and pigmentation problems.

The resurfacing can be local or full-face. Common smaller areas for resurfacing are: around the eyes (peri-ocular) and around the mouth (peri-oral). CO2 laser is particularly useful for improving the look of vertical wrinkles on the top lip. Fine lines disappear, while deeper lines are softened.

Laser is a high energy light beam which causes no bleeding and can be adjusted to permit a precise depth of resurfacing. It vaporizes and removes the top layers of 'old' skin, making way for 'new' skin that is smoother and more even in texture and color.

As well as removing a layer of skin the treatment heats the skin to tighten it. CO2 laser resurfacing can be performed in fractional mode (small columns of laser energy are fired into the skin, leaving some untreated skin) which reduces healing times, or in non-fractional mode, which has greater downtime.

The process of skin rejuvenation and facial skin tightening with this laser can be gradual. Patients can choose to have smaller doses and several treatments (up to four) or fewer treatments using higher doses.

Carbon dioxide laser resurfacing is performed while patients are under local anesthesia and mild sedation. It is a 'walk-in, walk-out' procedure with no need for hospitalization. It does, however, require some recovery 'down time' afterwards.

Immediately after the procedure the patient feels a sensation reminiscent of mild sunburn. The doctor prescribes antibiotics to be taken for the week following the procedure, to prevent bacterial infection.

The superficial layers of the skin will renew themselves within seven days. During this regeneration period the skin weeps. For the first three days fine, 'breathable' dressings should cover the treated area. After that a thin layer of gel should be applied for the remaining four days of the week.

After one week the new skin appears pink. Patients may wish to wear camouflaging makeup for up to three weeks, to disguise the pinkness. Eight days after the procedure, other people are unlikely to notice anything amiss with the patient's skin. New skin collagen formation continues for up to twelve months after the procedure.

Neither chemical peeling nor standard dermabrasion are as precise or as comfortable as laser. Protecting the skin by daily application of a broad spectrum sunscreen will prolong the results.

Potential problems include skin lightening. When deep wrinkles are vaporized to soften them, some pigment cells in the skin are also destroyed. As a result, the skin may look somewhat lighter.

Some names of carbon dioxide laser resurfacing devices include: 'Fractional CO2 Laser'.

Infrared Laser Skin Tightening

Infrared laser facial skin tightening is a non-ablative procedure that involves deep dermal heating of the dermis. When combined with other non-ablative procedures it can also improve conditions such as dyschromia (significant variation in skin color).

This treatment delivers a broad spectrum of infrared light which heats up the water content of the skin, causing the surrounding collagen to contract and tighten. Over the following months the body produces new collagen to further tighten the skin.

Infrared laser is not designed to treat large areas of loose or baggy skin, such as the kind that occurs after rapid, major weight-loss. That kind of skin is best treated with surgery.

Infrared is suitable for treating small areas of sagging skin on the abdomen (e.g. post pregnancy tummy), thighs and underarms and to tone, lift and tighten skin on the face and neck. Results vary significantly between individuals and some patients say they notice no improvement.

Some trade names of infrared facial skin tightening include Titan®.

Ultrasound Skin Tightening

Ultrasound facial skin tightening claims to 'shrink-wrap' your face from the inside, tightening sagging skin and triggering the growth of new collagen.

Alice Hart-Davis writes:

'It's loved by a host of stars including 'Friends' actress Courteney Cox ... Even the notoriously hard-to-please U.S. health watchdog, the Food and Drug Administration, likes [the treatment], deeming it the only non-invasive procedure to lift the skin on the neck, chin and brow.

'Unlike lasers, which zap the surface of the skin, [ultrasound facial skin tightening] uses ultrasound waves to heat something called the SMAS (superficial muscular aponeurotic system), the muscle-like layer of tissue under the skin.'[40]

When the SMAS muscle layer is heated, it contracts and tightens, which is the same effect produced by cosmetic surgeons when they suture the SMAS during a facelift procedure. Heating the tissue also stimulates the skin's production of new collagen, which continues during the following months.

Ultrasound treatment takes less than an hour. There is no recovery 'downtime' needed afterwards, because the effects take place below the skin's surface.

Following an ultrasound session, the patient's skin may look slightly red. This coloring normally fades in less than an hour. There is very little discomfort afterward; perhaps only a feeling of slight stiffness. It takes several months for the full results to become apparent.

Trade names of ultrasound skin tightening include Ultherapy®.

---

40   'The world's most AGONISING facial '. Alice Hart-Davis. Daily Mail Australia, Published: 09:55 AEST, 18 March 2013

FACE THERAPY: PRESERVING YOUR SKIN'S NATURAL TIGHTNESS

Our skin's elasticity decreases as we age, however there are some simple ways to delay this process and prolong the skin's firmness. These include losing weight gradually, drinking sufficient water, getting good nutrition and pampering your skin.

Avoid losing weight rapidly

Crash diets and excessive exercising can make your body rapidly shed both muscle and fat, resulting in a significant impact on your skin. If you lose muscle, the supportive underlying structure that holds skin against your body starts to shrink. Fat keeps the skin stretched out and if you lose it quickly the skin does not have time to snap back into place. As a general rule, aim to lose no more than ½–1 kilogram of fat per week. Ensure that you exercise regularly and include weight lifting in your workout, to avoid losing lean muscle.

If your skin does begin to look loose and saggy after you've lost weight, there's no need to worry because eventually, over time, it will shrink to fit your new, svelte shape.

However, if you are an older person, with decreased skin elasticity, this tightening may be minimal. Even in young people, skin tightening can take up to two years. To help your skin to stay elastic, follow these guidelines:

Drink plenty of water

Dried-out skin is less elastic. Try to consume at least two liters of water per day. This can be in the form of drinks and/or from watery foods such as soups.

Eat well

Your skin needs to obtain the building blocks to make collagen and elastin. Foods that contain the necessary vitamins, minerals and proteins for building collagen and elastin include tofu, beans, legumes, seeds, cottage cheese, nuts and fish.

Pamper your skin

Nourish your skin by regularly applying creams containing vitamins C, E and A. These have been proven to help to hydrate the skin and promote collagen and elastin production. See also page 273.

Exfoliate once or twice a week to remove dead skin cells and increase the skin's blood circulation. See "Exfoliation" on page 240.

Avoid air pollution and harmful chemicals such as sulfates and chlorine, which may be found in some detergents, soaps, shampoos and dishwashing liquids. Read the labels carefully and wear gloves when handling chemicals.

Ultraviolet rays can damage the skin so stay out of the sun and tanning salons.

Keep baths and showers tepid—not too hot.

FACE THERAPY: DERMAL FILLERS

Dermal fillers are substances that are injected into the skin to fill out, hydrate, augment or highlight areas of the face that have become saggy and wrinkled due to sun damage and aging. They can give you a fresher look, and result in a more youthful appearance. Wrinkles can be filled with a variety of substances, including collagen, hyaluronic acid, and other synthetic compounds. Some trade names of dermal fillers include Restylane®, Radiesse®, Juvederm®, Perlane® and ArteFill®.

Types of dermal fillers

There are two main types of dermal fillers: hydration boosters and volumizers. Both of them 'plump up' the skin in different ways. Many dermal filling substances perform both duties simultaneously.

Hydration boosting dermal fillers: Also known as 'hydration boosting', 'deep skin hydration' or 'hydroboosting' dermal fillers, these compounds are designed to treat the overall condition of your skin by improving skin tone, hydration and elasticity. They are best used to treat the whole face, neck and décolletage, to accentuate the cheek bones and to fill out the backs of the hands. Depending on the product used, the results of these injections can last from 6 months to 2 years.

Volumizing dermal fillers: These fillers are primarily designed to plump up and add fullness to smaller areas, such as the lips. Learn more by reading the section on volumizing dermal fillers (page 162).

Temporary (medium term) dermal fillers

All dermal fillers are, strictly speaking, temporary; that is, they are eventually absorbed into the body. Most dermal fillers last for a relatively short time–generally up to 18 months. These may be known as 'temporary'.

Trade names of temporary or 'medium term' fillers include Juvéderm®, Restylane®, Perlane®, Prevelle®, Teosyal®, Galderma Emervel® and Macrolane®.

Semi-permanent/permanent dermal fillers

Longer-lasting fillers (called 'permanent', 'semi-permanent' or 'long-acting' fillers) are also available.

Trade names of semi-permanent/permanent dermal fillers include Radiesse®, Sculptra®, ArteFill®, Dermatech Dermalive®, Hydrelle® (formerly known as Elevess), and Juvéderm® and Volbella®.

FACE THERAPY: HYDRATING DERMAL FILLERS

Benefits of hydrating dermal fillers

The skin's natural, youthful content of hyaluronic acid (one of the main components of the dermis) declines, over time, due to factors such as wind and sun damage, pollution, smoking, hormonal fluctuations and the natural process of aging. In particular, the skin of the face, neck, décolletage and hands becomes drier and more susceptible to showing wrinkles and lines.

Having properly hydrated skin is vital to looking good. Topically applied lotions and creams can offer only mild, short-term results. Hydrating dermal fillers can provide a more noticeable, long-lasting improvement. They replenish hyaluronic acid beneath the skin. After treatment the skin recovers much of its youthful radiance, tone and elasticity.

Hydrating dermal fillers are generally made of the skin hydrating agent hyaluronic acid (HA), which attracts water when injected into the skin and hence firms and plumps the injected areas.

Non-animal based hyaluronic acid is used, to minimize the risk of allergy. This substance is biocompatible and biodegradable.

Cosmetic clinics offer a range of hydrating dermal filler treatments. In general, treatment programs involve about three sessions over the course of three months.

Areas that can be treated with hydrating dermal fillers include the face, nasolabial folds, lips, cheeks, chin, the glabella (between the eyes), nose, acne scarring, jawline/jowls, temples, orbital rims (eye area), tear troughs, brow, earlobes, backs of hands, neck, and décolletage.

Micro-injections of hydrating dermal fillers

Some clinics offer treatments involving superficial micro-injections of hyaluronic acid into the skin. These are sometimes known as 'hydrating textural treatments'.

Micro-injection treatment involves several superficial injections into the skin, spaced 0.4–0.8 inches (1–2 cm) apart. Each session usually covers one area–for example the décolletage–and takes approximately 45 minutes. The procedure is performed with local anesthesia to reduce any discomfort. After the treatment, your esthetician will apply ice and firmly massage the treated area.

The hyaluronic acid is sometimes injected into the face using a 'threading' process. This is designed to effect a subtle lift in the lower face and, on completion of the course of treatments, help to improve the appearance of jowling.

Afterwards there may be some mild swelling in the treated area. This usually resolves within 24—48 hours. Any bruising will disappear completely within 1—10 days. Light makeup can be applied to conceal any bruising that may arise.

Skin texture is noticeably improved, right from the very first session. To maintain the results, repeat the treatment 2–3 times per year. Maintenance treatments can be less frequent after the first couple of years, especially if you combine hydrating dermal fillers with other rejuvenating therapies. With each treatment your skin will become firmer and the appearance of fine lines and wrinkles will decrease. Nonetheless, any existing deep grooves and wrinkles on the face or neck may need extra treatment with a volumizing dermal filler.

Hydrating dermal fillers are a good way to improve the skin's texture and minimize the appearance of fine wrinkles around the mouth, lips and cheeks. Injections of hydrating dermal fillers can also prolong the benefits of volumizing dermal fillers by helping to seal them in.

Some brand names of hydrating dermal fillers include Juvederm® Hydrate®, Restylane® and Rejuven8 Cosmetix®.

FACE THERAPY: VOLUMIZING DERMAL FILLERS

There are four main types of volumizing dermal fillers, each of a different thickness. The thinner fillers are used to treat fine lines and fragile areas of the skin, while the thicker fillers are used in larger areas; to plump up the cheeks or contour the jawline, for example. Volumizing fillers work well in the treatment of wrinkles and lines such as the naso-labial folds (furrows that run from the nose to the outer corners of the mouth), 'marionettes' (grooves that run downwards from the corners of the mouth) and fine lines around the mouth.

Other areas that can be treated with volumizing dermal fillers include the lips, cheeks, chin, glabella (between the eyes), nose, acne scarring, jawline/jowls, temples, orbital rims (eye area), tear troughs, brow, earlobes, backs of hands, neck, and décolletage.

Areas that benefit from volumizing dermal fillers

Forehead wrinkles. These are sometimes called 'worry lines'. They appear between the eyebrows and the hairline.

Frown lines. Frown lines between the eyebrows can be successfully smoothed out with volumizing dermal fillers.

Droopy eyebrows. As we age, our skin sags–especially the delicate skin around and above the eyes. Volumizing dermal fillers, skillfully injected, can lift this area.

Crows' feet. Many people do not mind having fine, crinkly lines of expression at the outer corners of the eyes, but when they become very indented they can mar our appearance.

Tear troughs. 'Tear troughs' are the curved indentations in the skin beneath our eyes, which can make our eyes look 'pouchy' or 'baggy'.

Bunny lines. These are tiny creases that appear along the sides of the nose. They are particularly obvious when you crinkle your nose, and they tend to get worse as you age.

Naso-labial folds. The grooves that run from the outer edges of the nostrils to the outer corners of the lips can be filled out with volumizing dermal fillers.

Hollow cheeks. As we get older, we lose fat from our cheeks. Instead of looking rounded and youthful, they become hollow-looking. This is called 'facial lipoatrophy'.

Marionettes. 'Oral commissures', the lines than droop from the outer corners of the mouth, are sometimes called 'marionettes'. This is because of their resemblance to the jaw-joints on the faces of ventriloquists' puppets. Marionettes can make our faces look sad, even when we feel happy. Volumizing dermal fillers provide a good solution.

Sagging jowls. Our cheeks lose fat as we age, and our skin's collagen deteriorates, thereby losing its elasticity. These factors combine to produce the appearance of sagging jowls. Injections of volumizing dermal fillers can lift jowls and re-structure the face.

As we age, our facial volume decreases, chiefly due to a loss of some of the subcutaneous fat layer. If this fat loss occurs in the sides of your chin that are sometimes called the 'prejowl area', then drooping jowls and a slight double chin may appear. To try to correct this with liposuction could cause more problems. The solution is to replenish the lost volume with injections of fat ("Fat transfer" on page 149) or volumizing dermal fillers.

Mental crease. Yes, 'mental crease'! It's a funny term for the little dip between the lower lip and the chin. It gets its name from the 'mentalis' muscle, which is a paired central muscle of the lower lip, situated at the tip of the chin.

Vertical lip lines. When you purse your lips you will see these lines appear. In older people, the lines can become permanent wrinkles.

Thin lips. Lips in both men and women reach their maximum volume in young adulthood. For many people, the lips begin shrinking between the ages of 30 and 40. Thin lips can make a person look older than their years. Studies show that women who have fuller and firmer lips are seen as younger than they really are. Angelina Jolie's bee-stung lips or Scarlett Johansson's pout may not be what you are looking for, but volumizing dermal fillers can certainly give you fuller lips.

Sagging mouth corners. Like 'marionettes', drooping skin at the outer corners of the mouth can make you look sad. Skilful injectors can plump up these areas. It's amazing what a difference a 'happy mouth' can make to your looks! Singer Avril Lavigne provides a good example of a natural 'happy mouth'. Even when she's not smiling, the corners of her mouth are turned up.

Ill-defined jaw line. As our cheeks droop, the fat that once sat beneath our cheekbones starts to hang around the lower jaw (mandible). The clean, sculpted jawline of youth gives way to a pudgy, formless appearance. Dermal fillers, properly injected, can help to rectify this.

Turkey neck. A wattle of loose skin flapping beneath one's chin conveys an elderly look. Sagging skin on the neck can be plumped out with dermal fillers.

FACE THERAPY: JAWLINE, NECK AND JOWLS REJUVENATION

Jawline and jowls

Sagging skin and wrinkles on the face are some of the most obvious signs of age. As we grow older poor facial muscle tone, loss of skin elasticity and facial volume, saggy skin, weight loss or weight gain, genetics, sleeping positions, repetitive mouth movements and bad habits like smoking can lead to the appearance of 'jowls'. Our facial fat pads age and droop, the face loses roundness, and we can end up with areas of facial skin or facial fat that have descended to hang along or below the jaw line. A once attractive triangular face has now turned into a square face. The firm, youthful jawline is replaced with soft, irregular flesh, and the new jowly face can make people look older and overweight.

Until recently, the only ways we could fight the effects of time on the jawline and jowls involved surgical facelifts, which often resulted in an unnatural, 'stretched' appearance.

Neck and décolletage

The neck is also an important area to rejuvenate, because your age is often judged by the appearance of your neck. The neck is subject to a number of degenerative changes such as loss of collagen and elastin and accumulation of fat. External factors such as wind, pollution and ultraviolet radiation play a major part. The neck and the décolletage area are particularly prone to premature aging because these are areas of increased sun exposure.

Traditionally, neck rejuvenation has been performed surgically to help to reposition lax skin, decrease wrinkles and reduce redundant fatty tissues. Non-surgical procedures can also address the skin texture of the neck and décolletage, whereas surgical procedures are unable to address this issue. Non-surgical jawline and neck rejuvenation can involve minimally invasive procedures with little or no downtime.

A variety of low-cost techniques can rejuvenate the skin and underlying tissues in the neck, jaw and jowls. The most important initial step is to block further sun-damage applying sunscreen, every day, on the neck, décolletage and hands, and not only the face.

SURGICAL JAWLINE, NECK AND JOWLS REJUVENATION

Surgical neck lift and treating vertical neck (platysmal) bands.

Skin laxity of the neck is best treated with plastic surgery. Non-surgical methods have attempted to emulate the results of surgery, but have so far been unsuccessful. For people with moderate amounts of loose skin and fatty pockets around the neck, surgery or minimally invasive surgery (such as 'thread weaving') is recommended.

Surgical neck lifts are performed while the patient is under general anesthesia. The surgeon makes one incision in front of the ear lobe, which curves around and ends behind the ear. He or she then makes a second, tiny cut in the crease between the under-surface of the chin and the neck, where any scars will be well hidden. Usually liposuction will be performed through these incisions, to remove excess neck fat, after which the neck skin will be separated from the underlying platysma muscle.

This muscle is then stitched together in the center, to enhance the shape of the neck in the vertical direction. This corrects the condition known as 'platysmal bands', which is the appearance of vertical, rope-like bands on the front of aging necks.

The outer edges of the muscle are also sutured and lifted up behind the ear to make a horizontal sling, which tightens the neck under the chin. The skin then repositioned over the muscle and tightened. Any excess loose skin is cut off, after which the incisions are closed.

Thread Lifting/Suture Lifting: Thread lifting is also known as suture lifting and subdermal thread lifting. This is a method of lifting the skin by placing a suture under the skin to pull the skin tight. Trade names include Contour® threads, Silhouette® threads, Aptos® threads, Featherlift®).

Liposuction: Excess neck fat is often treated with liposuction (see 'Liposuction' page 178). This is the most effective means of removing fat from under the chin and around the neck. It can be done under local anesthetic with or without sedation, and usually takes about two hours to perform. There is usually some retraction and tightening of neck skin, too, after liposuction.

Removal of jowl fat

As we age the 'buccal fat pad', an area of deep fat in the cheeks, droops into the jowl area.

Liposuction: The buccal fat pad can be removed to help define the cheekbones and decrease lower cheek volume in some patients. Careful consideration is highly recommended though, because facial fat can make faces look soft and relatively youthful; a gaunt face makes people look old. Consider dermal fillers as an alternative. Any facial liposuction should be done very sparingly, with a very small cannula to avoid bumps and dimples and other irregularities. Liposuction of the jowls can be performed under local anesthesia. Jowl liposuction is a delicate procedure, so seek a consultation with an extensively experienced surgeon.

Severe loose skin and fatty pockets

Surgery and laser: In the event the patient suffers from both severe loose skin and fatty pockets around the jawline and neck, the doctor may suggest the patient undertake a combination of both laser skin tightening and surgery,

MINIMALLY INVASIVE JAWLINE, NECK & JOWLS REJUVENATION

Neck wrinkles

'Horizontal neck bands' are creases in the skin of the neck caused by movement of the neck which creases the skin over time. These and other neck wrinkles can be treated in a number of ways.

Muscle relaxant injections. Horizontal neck bands can be treated with immobilizing wrinkle relaxing injections such as Botox, although the success of this procedure is low. (See page 183).

Dermal Fillers. A more effective treatment for neck wrinkles uses fillers. Depending on the size of the wrinkle, an appropriate dermal filler can be injected into the lines to help fill them out. See our 'volumizing dermal fillers' section (page 162).

Radiofrequency Therapies. Fine lines and wrinkles can also be treated with radiofrequency skin therapy (page 230).

Neck fat

Laser Therapy. The ideal candidate for laser fat removal and skin tightening of the neck is a person in good health, with an average body weight, who is unable to remove the stubborn fat deposits in and around the neck. With this treatment, fat deposits that are resistant to planned diets and workouts can be successfully removed. (See page 206).

Vertical neck bands

Vertical neck bands or 'platysmal bands' are caused by changes in the platysma muscle. This is the band of musculature that stretches from the collar bone to the jawline. Look into a mirror and clench your teeth hard: on your neck and beneath your jaw you will probably see the cord-like effects of your platysma muscle contracting. This muscle, over time, can separate into bands which may look aesthetically unpleasing. People who do a lot of 'sit-up' exercises are at greater risk of developing these bands.

Muscle relaxants. Just like horizontal neck bands, vertical neck bands can be treated with immobilizing wrinkle relaxing injections such as Botox. This may help flatten to them. Anti-wrinkle injections can also be injected into the areas where bands are not present, to help reduce the downward pull of the platysma muscle on the face. This can sometimes produce the effect of a 'lift' in the face.

Skin discoloration (sun damage and pigmentation)

Sun damage can cause skin pigmentation, which appears as brown patches. Red and scaly patches on the skin may be pre-cancerous lesions called solar (actinic) keratosis. Sun exposure is cumulative, and over time, these sorts of lesions may appear— especially on fairer skin types. The treatment of solar keratosis is not only cosmetic, but also preventative, because pre-cancerous lesions should be removed immediately. Other forms of skin discoloration include 'Poikiloderma of Civatte' [41].

---

41   *Poikiloderma of Civatte' is a skin condition which appears as reddish brown discoloration on sides of the neck, usually on both sides. The area that is shaded by the chin is usually free of the discoloration. This condition is more common with women than men and more commonly effects middle-aged to elderly women. Poikiloderma is exacerbated by UV exposure, but the underlying cause is not known. Perfumes and various cosmetics have been implicated, as well as hormonal causes like low oestrogen levels. People with a family history of poikiloderma as well as fair-skinned individuals are more likely to develop this condition. Avoidance of potential causes of poikiloderma such as perfumes, UV radiation, and various cosmetics is the first step in treating poikiloderma. This skin condition can be treated effectively with the Pulsed dye laser or Gemini laser. 'Poikiloderma' is basically a change of the skin due to dilation of the blood vessels in the neck. "Civatte" was the French dermatologist who first identified it in the 1920s. (Source: Poikiloderma of Civatte, Medscape, Author: Lana H Hawayek, MD., Chief Editor: Dirk M Elston, MD. Undated article retrieved December 2014.)*

Laser: Skin discoloration, especially brown pigmentation, can be treated effectively with a Pulsed Dye Laser or Gemini® Laser. This helps to reduce the pigmentation and close off any superficial capillaries causing the redness. The wavelengths from these lasers are specifically attracted to the capillaries and pigmentation, and hence normal skin is relatively unaffected. The Gemini® laser emits a green wavelength of light that is attracted to the brown pigmentation on the neck and helps to break it down. Lasers such as the Medlite® laser and ruby laser can also be used to treat brown spots on the neck and chest area.

Peels: The tissues of the neck are usually thinner and more sensitive than that of the face, and need to be treated more cautiously. Chemical peels may be used to help exfoliate dead skin cells and reduce pigmentation and solar damage. Skin care containing retinoic acid or hydroquinone can also help, but can be very irritating in this area in comparison to their effect on the face.

Topical applications: Skin-lightening creams are available for hyper-pigmentation disorders.

Photodynamic Therapy: Photodynamic therapy is particularly effective at treating solar keratosis. Sun damage and pigmentation can also be treated with photodynamic therapy.

Combination discoloration, wrinkles, and skin laxity:

Plasma skin regeneration is another method of resurfacing the neck. It uses plasma energy to decrease pigmentation, and also has the added advantage of reducing wrinkles and tightening skin.

Only the lower energy settings can be used on the neck with plasma however, and therefore a number of treatment sessions may be required to achieve the optimal results.

Drooping jowls

Jowls can be treated by a number of surgical or non-surgical procedures. Some non-invasive treatments include acupuncture, microcurrent, and suction cup massage, or combinations thereof.

Microcurrent Jowl Removal. This technique is claimed to tighten 'turkey neck' throat, achieve smooth and wrinkle-free skin and remove jowls and pouches. See "microcurrent cosmetic rejuvenation" on page 222.

Acupuncture Jowl Removal. Acupuncturists claim that the skilled use of acupuncture needles can 'remove blockages in the free flow of energy' on the hands, feet, scalp and face, and can help reduce wrinkles and firm skin. They suggest facial acupuncture as a rejuvenation therapy for people over the age of 35. There are acupuncture techniques that specifically target issues such as loose jowls, double chins, deep wrinkles, under-eye bags and droopy eyelids. It is recommended that patients attend twelve sessions for best results.

Suction cup massage. With this treatment, glass suction tubes designed for the face are placed on the skin. The esthetician uses them to rhythmically create a vacuum. It is claimed that this suction lifts, tones, and plumps muscles; softens wrinkles; removes toxins; increases elastin and collagen; boosts lymphatic drainage and increases circulation. It is painless and leaves no marks. Silicone facial massage cupping sets are available on the market for home use.

Note that the efficacy of suction cup massage has not been proven.

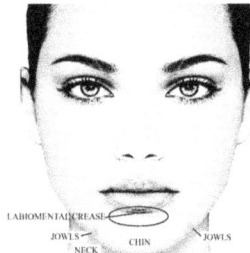

Neck skin laxity
Minimally-invasive treatments for skin laxity of the neck include:

Laser Skin Tightening. Laser skin tightening is used to improve the appearance of 'turkey necks' and 'double chins' without the need to remove excess skin. This procedure is suitable for people with small amounts of loose skin and fatty pockets in the neck. Laser skin tightening removes small fatty deposits while tightening and improving the quality of the surrounding skin. Practitioners advertise it as a 'walk in, walk out procedure' that takes only half an hour, with no recovery time needed and without the scars associated with surgery. See "Skin Therapy: laser skin therapies" on page 206.

Subdermal Laser Threading
For patients that suffer solely from loose skin around the neck area, a subdermal laser threading procedure is more successful.

Radiofrequency Skin Tightening. Machines like the Thermage®, Accent® fat blaster, Titan®, and Refirme ST®, can use radiofrequency to heat the skin, thereby stimulating collagen production and tightening the skin. The effects are usually variable and subtle. See page 230.

Ultrasound Skin Tightening. This is a non-surgical procedure which stimulates collagen production and thereby improves skin elasticity. Brand names include Ulthera®. See page 244.

Infrared Skin Tightening. This is a non-surgical, non-ablative procedure using red light. Infrared skin treatment can reduce the appearance of wrinkles, remodel skin, treat acne and acne scars, improve skin texture, and increase collagen and elastin. See page 211.

Carbon Dioxide Laser Resurfacing. Fractional carbon dioxide laser treatments can be used for resurfacing the neck and to help with skin texture, wrinkles and to tighten neck skin. See "Laser Skin Therapies', page 206.

Microneedling Radiofrequency Skin Tightening. Skin needling, also known as 'collagen induction therapy' (CIT), employs the body's own natural healing response to produce more collagen, resulting in skin rejuvenation and reduction of wrinkles. See page 231.

Microcurrent Facials stimulate healthy collagen remodeling inside the skin, to tighten sagging skin and naturally fill in wrinkles at the jaw line, around the eyes, at the brow line and around the mouth and cheeks to lift sagging jowls. See page 222.

Plasma Skin Regeneration can successfully treat early jowling and loosening skin. See page 225.

Vacuum Suction Facials can also stimulate healthy collagen remodeling inside the skin, tightening lax skin and filling in wrinkles. See page 248.

Wrinkle Relaxing Injections. Wrinkle relaxing injections can provide a non-surgical 'lower face lift'. They are used to elevate sagging jowls, soften marionette lines and sharpen the jaw line. This effect is achieved by relaxing part of the tight-pulling platysma muscle, which contributes to sagging around the jawline and thus exaggerates the jowls. Once the platysma is no longer pulling downwards, muscles on the upper face can lift the lower face, creating a more defined jaw line. The procedure should be carried out by skilled clinicians trained in the exact placement and dosage that are crucial for optimum results.

As with most treatments using wrinkle injections, the results last for around three months, there is no recovery period and patients can return to normal duties immediately. Trade names of wrinkle relaxing injection protocols for the neck include the 'Nefertiti Lift'.

NECK SKIN TAGS

A skin tag is a tiny, harmless pouch of skin hanging off the underlying skin, usually on the end of a slender stalk. Skin tags generally form in places where there is friction from clothing or skin from another part of the body. Such places may include the groin, underarms, neck, and chest. We are not born with skin tags. They tend to form as we get older, and in fact around 25% of adults have them. Because they are harmless, they only require treatment if you find their presence distressing. Three forms of treatment are common:

Surgery for skin tags—Skin tags can be removed by cutting them off with a sharp, sterile blade, scissors, or radiowave surgery; by freezing them off with liquid nitrogen; or by burning them off with electric cautery. It is recommended to have these procedures done in the doctor's clinic. If skin tags are growing on the eyelids, your doctor will also consult an ophthalmologist (eye doctor).
While very small skin tags can be removed without any anesthetic, larger ones require the use of local anesthesia via injections or a topical anesthetic cream.

Gemini laser for skin tags—This laser can remove small skin tags. Sometimes more than one treatment is needed to get a good result. Gemini laser is recommended for patients who have numerous small skin tags, as the laser can be directed accurately at the lesion without affecting the surrounding skin.

Self-treatments for skin tags—Some people tie a piece of strong thread or dental floss around the stalks of small skin tags and wait for the tag to fall off. This process may take several days.

FACE THERAPY: NATURAL WAYS TO KEEP JAWLINE, NECK AND JOWLS LOOKING YOUNG

Sleeping positions can reduce jowls

You may not consider sleeping in the same position every night as a cause of sagging jowls. However, sleeping on your side night after night, pressing your face into the pillow, can really affect the skin of the chin and cheeks.

The American Academy of Dermatology says that the jawlines of people who sleep on their backs sag less than those of people who sleep with their faces pushed against a pillow.

There are several 'anti-wrinkle' pillows on the market specifically designed to prevent you from sleeping on your face. Trade names include (but are not limited to) 'Juverest® Sleep Wrinkle Pillow' and 'Vasseur® Anti Wrinkle Beauty Pillow'.

Sunscreen

The skin of the neck and décolletage is likely to be more frequently exposed to UV radiation, and this causes progressive degenerative changes in the skin. Prevent further sun damage by daily application of sunscreen to exposed skin—not just on the face but also on the neck, décolletage, and backs of hands.

Quit smoking

Smoking cigarettes speeds up the normal aging process of our skin, causing wrinkling and sagging. The nicotine in cigarettes produces narrowing of the blood vessels near the skin surface. This restricts blood flow to your skin. With less blood flow, your skin doesn't get the oxygen and important nutrients, such as vitamin A, which provide protection from sun damage. Many of the more than 4,000 chemicals in tobacco smoke also damage collagen and elastin, the fibrous proteins that give your skin its strength and elasticity. Wrinkles and facial sag develop prematurely in smokers, and this can contribute to jowling.

Exercise to tone the platysmal muscle

One common exercise—sit-ups—should actually be *avoided*, if you wish to keep unsightly 'platysmal bands' at bay. However you can practice other neck exercises to keep the platysma muscle in good condition. Movement increases muscle strength, flexibility and tone, so exercising all the muscles of the lower face, jaw and neck will engage the platysma muscle group. This can help to retain the youthful lift of your neck and jawline. Even simply tilting your head slowly from side to side or front to back will strengthen the platysmal muscle. Such easy exercises can be performed several times a day. Here are some examples:

The Tilted Goldfish.

Stand up straight and tilt your head back as far as it will comfortably go. Now, slowly open and close your mouth. Repeat 10 times. Perform this exercise twice a day until you become accustomed to it, then practice more often.

The Bulldog.

Holding your head straight, push up your lower jaw until the lower teeth touch the upper lip. Repeat this 10 times. Do this exercise up to four times a day.

For an extra boost slowly tilt your head back, still holding this position, until you can see the ceiling. Remain in this position for 8—0 seconds, then relax.

The Tongue Resistor

Lift up your chin and place the tips of your middle and index fingers underneath, on the soft tissue beneath the chin. Press down your tongue against your lower jaw until you feel the pressure on your fingertips. This creates resistance against the platysma muscle. Hold this position for 10 seconds before relaxing the tongue. Wait another 10 seconds then repeat four more times.

The Haka.

Sit bolt-upright with your shoulders aligned with your hips and your spine as vertical as possible. Keep your head pointed straight ahead and your chin level.

Now, without moving your head, open your mouth as wide as you can without hurting yourself. Thrust out your tongue and try to touch your chin with it. Hold this position for 5 seconds and then relax. Wait for 2 seconds before repeating this process ten times.

The "Scuse Me While I Kiss the Sky'.

Assume the same starting position as for 'The Haka'. Slowly tilt your chin toward the ceiling, then purse your lips and stretch your neck as if you were trying to kiss the sky.

Hold this position for 5 seconds and then relax. Wait a couple of seconds and repeat. Repeat 10 times per session.

Variation: Instead of kissing the sky, chew it. Pop a piece of gum in your mouth and chew, while looking up with your head tilted back.

The Almost-a-Situp.

Lie flat on your back on a relatively flat surface – either a yoga mat, the floor or your bed. You must not be using a pillow.

Lift only your head. Tuck your chin under and continue to lift your head while keeping your shoulders flat against the surface. Try to touch your chest with your chin.

Hold this position for 6 seconds, then relax. After a couple pf seconds repeat the exercise. Ten repetitions per session should suffice.

Note: with 'sit-ups' you would be lifting your shoulders and torso off the floor. Avoid this!

ⓘ FACE THERAPY: LIPOSUCTION

Liposuction, also known as lipoplasty, liposculpture, suction lipectomy or simply lipo, is a cosmetic surgical procedure that removes fat from beneath the skin. Patients may be placed under general, regional, or local anesthesia for liposuction.

Areas of the face and neck where liposuction may be performed are the face, neck, jowls, chin and throat. It is not so much the amount of fat removed that can improve a person's appearance, as how well the facial contouring has been performed. Skilful liposuction can enhance the facial features, particularly beneath the chin.

As with any surgery there are certain risks, beyond the temporary and minor side effects.

Techniques of liposuction include:

- *Suction-assisted liposuction (SAL).* This is the traditional method, in which the surgeon inserts a small cannula (thin tube) into the layer of fat beneath the skin. The cannula is attached to a vacuum device. The surgeon maneuvers the tube through the fat layer, using it to mechanically break up the fat cells so that they can be sucked out of the body.

- *Internal ultrasound-assisted liposuction (UAL)*, during which the ultrasonic energy is applied through a specialized cannula inserted into the tissues. The broken-down fat is then extracted by traditional liposuction. Trade names include VASER, which stands for 'Vibration Amplification of Sound Energy at Resonance'. Vaser liposuction is also called VASERlipo.

- *External ultrasound-assisted liposuction (EUA, XUAL or EUAL).* This technique involves ultrasound being delivered through the skin without any surgical incisions; after which traditional surgical liposuction is carried out. The idea is that pre-treatment with ultrasound breaks down the fat and makes it easier to remove.

- *Power-assisted liposuction (PAL)*. With this technique the surgeon uses a powered, mechanized cannula, so that it is not necessary to use only muscular force to break up the fat. In other respects PAL is similar to standard SAL.

- *Twin-cannula (assisted) liposuction (TCAL or TCL)*

- *Water-assisted liposuction (WAL)*. WAL employs a slender, fan-shaped water jet, which breaks up the fat tissue so that it can be more easily extracted by a suction cannula.

- *Laser assisted liposuction*. A laser is used to disrupt and liquefy the fat before it is removed.

Liposuction is used more often to treat the body than the face. For a more in-depth discussion of this procedure, read the companion book in this series, *Ultimate Beauty 2: Hair, Body and Smile.*

FACE THERAPY: MESOTHERAPY

Mesotherapy is a minimally invasive, non-surgical technique which was originally invented to relieve the discomfort and pain of inflammatory skin conditions such as eczema and psoriasis. It involves micro-injections of compounds such as fat-dissolving phosphatidyl-choline, plant extracts, anesthetics, amino acids, vitamins, minerals, homeopathic remedies and enzymes into the mesoderm, or middle layer of skin. The ingredients of this 'cocktail' vary depending on the patient's individual requirements.

Mesotherapy advocates claim that the technique can be used on the body to reduce pockets of unwanted fat on the hips, stomach and abdomen, outer and inner thighs, back, buttocks, knees, arms, waist and even hands. On the face, jawline, neck and décolletage it can be used to improve the appearance of wrinkles and lines, jowls and double chins, and fat pads beneath the eyes. It is also used for skin rejuvenation and may result in a slight improvement in the appearance of cellulite.

A topical anesthetic cream may be applied before treatment, and ice may be applied afterwards.

After treatment, patients can resume their normal activities immediately.

Potential side effects may include a sensation of burning or itching, temporary soreness, some bruising. These problems usually resolve by themselves within a few days. There may be a risk of swelling, infection, and irregular contours.

FACE THERAPY: NOSE RESHAPING

SURGICAL NOSE RESHAPING (RHINOPLASTY)
Rhinoplasty (a nose job), is a cosmetic surgical procedure for aesthetically enhancing the nose. The surgeon creates a functional, better-looking and facially proportionate nose by separating the nasal skin and the soft tissues from the nasal framework, correcting them as required, suturing the incisions, and applying either a nasal pack, a small plastic nose splint, or a stent, to immobilize the corrected nose to ensure the proper healing of the surgical incision.[42]

As with all surgeries there is a need for downtime during the healing process, and there may be associated risks and complications.

---

42   *Rhinoplasty. From Wikipedia, the free encyclopedia. Article retrieved November 2014.*

NON-SURGICAL NOSE RESHAPING

The nose is a very important facial feature. Even small improvements in the contour of the nose can improve the symmetry and beauty of the face, boosting self-image and confidence. Minor defects in the shape of the nose can be corrected by using nonsurgical nose reshaping procedures.

Non-surgical nose reshaping involves the injection of dermal fillers to achieve the desired contour of the nose. It is used to mold the bridge of the nose, enhance the shape and projection of the tip of the nose, even out any humps and correct minor defects that may have been caused by rhinoplasty. It has several advantages:

- It is minimally invasive.
- It has no recovery time and shows immediate improvement.
- The whole procedure takes only 30 minutes.
- It is more affordable.
- It is done under local anesthesia so you can interact with the cosmetic surgeon during the procedure to fine tune the desired results.
- The results are not permanent and can be redone if you are not happy with the results after its effect fades away.
- It can be used in place of revision rhinoplasty to correct small deformities without any complications.

Any bruising and swelling that occurs after the procedure will usually subside within two days. The results of nonsurgical nose reshaping are temporary and last for about two years. Repeated treatments are required for maintenance.

FACE THERAPY: ULTRASOUND FACE THERAPY

Ultrasound face therapy is a non-surgical procedure used to lift and tighten the muscles of the face, neck and brow. After treatment the full results may take a few months to appear. Ultrasound can also be used to reduce small pockets of fat in the jowls and to benefit the skin on your face, improving the look of fine lines and scar tissue.

See also our section on 'ultrasound skin therapy' (page 244) for further information.

Ultrasound as a non-surgical 'facelift'

The U.S. Food and Drug Administration (FDA) has approved an ultrasound treatment by the trade name of Ultherapy. This treatment is said to tighten and lift the muscles and skin of the neck, face and eyebrows. The Ulthera® device delivers ultrasound into the muscles and skin, heating them to stimulate collagen production in both deep and superficial tissue layers.

Ultrasound energy is able to penetrate deeper than any other form of energy used for cosmetic purposes. It passes deep into the SMAS layer of muscle that stretches across the neck and lower face. This is the very layer that surgeons tighten with sutures when they perform surgical facelifts. See also page 244.

One session usually suffices, though patients may need two.

Ultrasound for facial fat reduction

The effects of ultrasound on fat reduction have been well documented. Ultrasound is used to prepare the fat prior to liposuction and during the liposuction process. It breaks up and liquefies the fat so that it can be sucked out more easily. Both external ultrasound assistance (EUA, XUAL or EUAL) and ultrasonic assisted liposuction (UAL) are very successful.

Recently, ultrasound has also been used as the sole method of dissolving fat. In this procedure, saline fluid is injected into the area to be treated, and the ultrasound applied for five to eight minutes without liposuction. In even a few sessions, patients obtain noticeable improvement in areas of small fatty accumulations such as the jowls.

Note that ultrasound skin therapy alone does not correct sun damage; neither does it reduce hollows caused by age-related fat loss.

For these reasons it may be used in combination with other treatments, such as dermal fillers and laser resurfacing, or a chemical peel.

FACE THERAPY: WRINKLE RELAXING INJECTIONS

Most people have heard of an anti-wrinkle treatment called Botox®. It is one of a range of brand names for wrinkle relaxing injections. The active ingredients in these wrinkle relaxing injections are purified versions of the botulinum toxin A (BTX-A).

Botulinum toxin is a protein and neurotoxin produced by the bacterium *Clostridium botulinum.*

Injections of BTX-A, performed by trained clinician, are used to treat wrinkles. BTX-A works by paralyzing, or 'relaxing' the muscles we use in facial expressions, allowing the skin on top of those muscles to lie smooth and crease-free.

The effects of wrinkle relaxing injections generally last four to six months. As muscle paralysis gradually wears off, the lines and wrinkles begin to re-appear and you may wish to have them treated again. Over time, with regular treatments, lines and wrinkles may appear less severe because the underlying muscles are 'getting accustomed' to relaxing.

Wrinkle relaxing injections are useful for treating:
- Forehead frown lines
- Crows' feet
- Frown lines between the eyebrows
- Folds at the outer corners of the mouth
- 'Bunny' lines flanking the nose
- Sagging eyebrows

'Three forms of botulinum toxin type A (Botox®, Dysport® and Xeomin®) and one form of botulinum toxin type B (MyoBloc®) are available commercially for various cosmetic and medical procedures.'[43]

---

43   Source: *Wikipedia, the free encyclopedia. Article retrieved August 2014.*

Part 4:
Skin Therapy

SKIN THERAPY

The skin is the largest organ of the body, with a total area of about 1.8 square metres (20 square feet). Skin safeguards us from bacteria and other microorganisms, protects us from the elements, helps regulate body temperature, and allows the sensations of touch, heat, and cold.

Skin is composed of three layers:
- *The epidermis.* The outermost layer of skin, the epidermis furnishes a waterproof barrier and is responsible for our skin tone. It also houses cells called melanocytes, which produce the pigment 'melanin'. Melanin determines the color of our skin.
- *The dermis.* This lies beneath the epidermis. It comprises hair follicles and sweat glands, as well as tough connective tissue such as collagen and elastin fibers that provide skin with strength, toughness, elasticity and pliability,
- *The hypodermis.* This deeper tissue beneath the dermis is composed of fat and connective tissue.

As the body ages, the appearance and characteristics of the skin alter. The epidermis becomes thinner so blemishes become more visible, and collagen in the dermis is gradually lost which contributes to the formation of facial lines, sagging skin and wrinkles.

Balanced pH: The skin's own natural barrier, the 'acid mantle', performs most efficiently when it is slightly acidic, at a 5.5 pH balance. If it becomes too alkaline, the skin suffers from dryness and over-sensitivity. It may become prone to eczema and vulnerable to inflammation, ultimately leading to a breakdown of collagen and an increase in wrinkles and sagging.

Cosmetic skin therapy offers hope for treating issues such as:
- acne and acne scarring
- blackheads and whiteheads
- pigmentation, discoloration, pigmentation and vitiligo
- dry skin

- eczema and psoriasis
- enlarged pores
- scars, stretch marks and pock marks
- skin lesions
- unwanted tattoos
- sagging skin
- varicose veins, spider veins
- wrinkles

Skin therapies discussed in this section include:

* Chemical peels
* Cosmetic tattooing
* Dermabrasion and microdermabrasion
* Infra-red skin therapy
* Intense Pulsed Light (IPL)
* Laser skin therapy
* Low-level laser therapy (LLLT)
* Photodynamic therapy
* Plasma skin regeneration
* PRP injections
* Radiofrequency
* Radiowave surgery
* Skin needling
* Skin care formulations
* Topical applications of serums, lotions, creams etc.
* Vacuum suction
* Wrinkle paralysis injections, eg. Botox
* Radiofrequency
* Ultrasound

We also discuss a basic skin care kit for home use and provide some recipes for those who would like to make their own skin care preparations.

No matter which treatment you and your dermatologist, surgeon or esthetician choose, ensure that you receive all the information on what to expect and what is required of you before and after the procedure.

SKIN THERAPY: BASIC SKIN CARE KIT

Create your own Basic Skin Care Kit. For an essential anti-aging skin care pack, dermatologists recommend–

- A mild cleanser (to remove impurities and unclog pores).
- An antioxidant vitamin C serum worn during the day.[44]
- A moisturizer.
- A daily broad-spectrum sunscreen, SPF 15 to 30, (to protect skin from the aging effects of the sun).
- A retinol cream (derived from vitamin A) applied at night.

The bare minimum: If you wish to pare down your skin care kit and make it even more basic, you could simply use a cleanser, a moisturizer and a sunscreen.

The extended version with extras: If you wish to expand your skin care kit you could add toners, facial scrubs, chemical exfoliants, a comedones extractor, an electric face-cleansing/vacuuming/massaging/ exfoliating brush, a pigmentation-fading cream and cleansing/moistur- izing facial masks.

ABOUT SERUMS:

The purpose of facial serums is to allow nutrients to soak into the deeper skin layers that standard moisturizers are not able to reach.

---

44   *'Vitamin C is a potent antioxidant drug that can be used topically in der- matology to treat and prevent changes associated with photoaging. It can also be used for the treatment of hyperpigmentation.' Vitamin C in dermatology, Pumori Saokar Telang, Indian Dermatol Online J. 2013 Apr-Jun; 4(2): 143–146. doi: 10.4103/2229-5178.110593, PMCID: PMC3673383*

The molecules in serums are smaller than the molecules in moisturizers, so moisturizers cannot penetrate the skin as deeply as serums.

Serums are about skin nutrition while moisturizers are about adding moisture to the skin and keeping it there with a protective barrier.

There are many types of serums commercially available, including anti-aging serums, skin brightening serums and even acne preventative serums.

Serums contain high concentrations of certain active ingredients. These ingredients may be substances such as retinol (with a wide range of skin benefits), hyaluronic acid (to improve the look of lines and wrinkles), vitamin C (to brighten the skin and help fade pigmentation and age spots) or glycolic acid (to exfoliate the skin).

Serums can really benefit your skin. For example, when we consume vitamins in food, most of those vitamins are used throughout the whole body and only a tiny portion reaches the skin. When we apply vitamins directly to the skin via serums, however, the skin reaps all the benefits.

If you are to receive the full benefits of serums you must use them correctly and consistently. They should be applied after you cleanse your skin, but before you apply moisturizer.

Apply serums when your skin is still slightly damp from rinsing. As with cleansing and moisturizing, remember to cover your neck and upper chest when rubbing on the serum. After approximately four weeks of daily use, improvements in the skin's appearance become noticeable.

ABOUT TONERS:

Toners are really unnecessary, particularly if you cleanse your skin properly. In fact, some commercially available astringent toners can harm your skin by stripping away its natural oils.

Toners used to be touted as 'pore refining'; however, they do not in fact close the skin's pores because pores don't have their own muscles, so they are incapable of opening and closing. We recommend bypassing toners and saving your time and money for skin care products that really work.

AN OVERVIEW OF SKINCARE PRODUCTS:

All skincare (and haircare) products, whether synthetic, organic or a combination of both, contain some or all of the following ingredients in various forms and proportions:

- occlusives
- humectants
- emollients
- emulsifiers
- surfactants (used in hair shampoos)
- preservatives

Occlusives.

An occlusive is a barrier. Occlusives include such substances as petrolatum (petroleum jelly), paraffin, lanolin, lecithin, cocoa butter, mango seed butter, shea butter, and beeswax. These substances form a barrier layer on top of the skin that traps water inside the skin and prevents it from being lost when the skin is exposed to dry air or wind.

Emulsifying wax, used to stabilize skincare products, also acts as an occlusive.

White soft paraffin, also known as white petroleum jelly, is not an active ingredient as such, but works as an occlusive moisturizer by providing a layer of oil on the surface of the skin to prevent water evaporating.

Petrolatum has been shown in studies to be highly beneficial for the skin, despite claims to the contrary. Topical application of petrolatum can help the skin's outer layer recover from damage, reduce inflammation, and generally heal the skin.[45]

Substances such as zinc oxide and white petrolatum are occlusives that are used mostly to protect the skin against irritation.

Humectants.

Humectants are water-binding agents. They penetrate the outermost layer of the epidermis (the stratum corneum, which consists of dead cells) and draw water into the cells that lie beneath. This increases the skin's water-holding capacity and causes its surface to swell very slightly—thus temporarily making it appear smoother and more wrinkle-free. These water-binding agents are used to treat or prevent dry, rough, scaly, itchy skin and minor skin irritations.

Humectants include such substances as sorbitol, sodium hyaluronate, urea, propylene glycol, and sugars, and alpha hydroxy acids such as lactic/citric/glycolic acid.

Some examples of natural humectants are lecithin, sugar, panthenol (pro-vitamin B5), and vegetable glycerin.

Note to those who make their own skincare preparations: Glycerin should be used at a concentration of 3—10% in skincare formulations. More than that and it will draw moisture out of the skin instead of moisturizing it.

Emollients.

---

45   Source: *Acta Dermato-Venereologica, November–December 2000, pages 412–415.*

Emollients soften and moisturize the skin and decrease itching and flaking. They enter the gaps between rough or peeling skin cells, filling them up and smoothing the skin's surface.

Lanolin, mineral oil, and petrolatum are occlusive agents that also serve as emollients.

Numerous kinds and trade names of emollients exist, varying from watery lotions to viscous creams and ointments. The distinction between lotions, creams and ointments is the percentage of water to lipid (oil). Lotions contain the least amount of oil, while creams contain a moderate amount and ointments the most. The more oil, the creamier and thicker the texture. In general, a high oil content means the formulation is more effective and long-lasting, but some people find it less pleasant to use.

In moisturizers, the emollient ingredients may be oil-based or water-based. Oil-based emollients are richer and may absorb completely into the skin. This makes them ideal for people with dry skin which requires deep moisturizing. Water-based emollients, by contrast, are more lightweight and less sticky, which means they are perfect for those who have normal, oily or acne-prone skin.'[46]

Some examples of excellent natural skin emollients are jojoba oil, avocado oil, rosehip oil, argan oil, coconut oil, shea butter, cocoa butter, jojoba butters, vegetable glycerin, gamma linolenic acid (GLA), hydroxylated lecithin, sunflower seed oil, jojoba wax, caprylic/capric triglyceride extract derived from coconut, kukui nut oil, corn oil, grape seed oil, borage seed oil, safflower seed oil, evening primrose oil, mango seed butter, almond oil, apricot kernel oil and pumpkin seed extract.

Emulsifiers

The job of emulsifiers is to blend and bind ingredients which usually separate from one another. An emulsifier can either be a physical substance, like wax, or a physical action, like shaking a lotion to blend it.

---

46   Source: Karen Bruno on WebMD, Article retrieved November 2014.

Many people who make their own skincare products at home use emulsifying wax as a binder (or, for shampoos, BTMS-50 conditioning emulsifier).

Natural emulsifiers are obtained from certain leaves, nuts and berries. Some examples of natural emulsifiers are xanthan gum, quince seed, vegetable glycerin and plant waxes such as candelilla, carnauba, jojoba, and rice bran wax.

Surfactants

Surfactants, or 'surface-active-agents,' are compounds that act to dissolve oils and hold dirt in suspension so that it can be rinsed away. They are essential ingredients in skin cleansers and hair shampoos.

Natural saponins (foaming agents) are excellent in skin cleansers, shampoos and body washes because they clean the hair and skin very gently, without stripping away the natural oils. Some examples of natural surfactants are castile soap, soapwort, soapnuts, yucca extract, and quillaja bark extract. Note, however, that castile soap is very alkaline, which can adversely affect the skin's acid mantle ("acid mantle" on page 185) and cause problems.

Preservatives

Preservatives help prevent bacterial and fungal growth in skincare and other formulations. They give products a longer shelf life.

Rot and decay are natural processes in all organic materials. Even with preservatives, natural skincare products will eventually deteriorate and go rancid; this is normal.

Some examples of natural preservatives are bitter orange extract and grapefruit seed extract. Tea tree essential oil and thyme essential oil are also natural preservatives; however essential oils should not be used on the skin (see "Beware of essential oils" on page 257).

COMMERCIAL SKIN CARE PRODUCTS:

Cosmetics manufacturers generally use a lot of synthetic ingredients, because:

- Synthetics cost less than natural ingredients
- It is easy to obtain manufactured ingredients than natural ingredients
- They can be diluted with little effort

Because chemicals are relatively cheap, commercial skin care preparations do not have to cost a lot in order to do their job. You can go ahead and purchase the five basic skin care preparations from druggists, pharmacies, supermarkets, beauticians, day spas etc., or you can make your own.

It is not necessary to depend on manufactured ingredients to make highly effective skincare products. There are hundreds of natural ingredients that actually outclass synthetics in terms of performance, as well as being environmentally sound and sustainable.

HOME-MADE SKIN CARE FORMULATIONS

The recipes section (page 250) of this book includes the following:

Home-made Skin Cleansers
- Clay Skin Cleanser page 263
- Orris Root Powder Skin Cleanser page 265
- Chickpea Flour Skin Cleanser page 263
- Raw Organic Honey Skin Cleanser page 265
- Refreshing Skin Cleanser page 264
- Soothing Skin Cleanser page 264

Home-made Skin Serums
- Vitamin C Serum page 273
- Retinol Serum page 276
- Vitamin B and E Serum page 279

Home-made Skin Moisturizers

- Basic Moisturizer (with emulsifying wax) page 269
- Basic Moisturizer (without emulsifiers) page 271

Home-made Facial Peels
- AHA (citric & lactic acid) Facial Peel page 250
- BHA (salicylic acid) Facial Peel page 286

Home-made Sunscreen
- Basic Home-made Sunscreen page 294

Home-made Pore Refining Treatments
- Cucumber and Egg Pore Refining Mask page 288
- Simple Lemon Juice and Egg Pore Refining Treatment page 290

Home-made Skin Care: Skin Lightening Treatments
- Simple Lemon Juice Skin Lightener page 291
- Lemon Juice and Turmeric Skin Lightener page 291
- Simple Aloe Vera Skin Lightener page 291

Home-made Soothing Skin Spritzers
- Rose Flower Water page 259
- Hibiscus Flower Water page 262

Home-made Exfoliating Scrubs
- AHA (glycolic acid) Facial Peel/Scrub page 286
- Cleansing Skin Exfoliant page 283

Home-made Temporary Skin Tightening Masks
- Egg White Skin Tightening Mask page 294

SKIN THERAPY: CHEMICAL PEELS

Chemical peels are a procedure for rejuvenating the skin by inflicting controlled damage. They remove the top layers of skin to encourage collagen production, thereby improving sun-damaged skin, skin pigmentation problems, wrinkles, skin texture, and the general look of the skin.

Deeper chemical peels require stronger formulations. They are also associated with a larger number of unwanted side-effects and a longer recovery time, but the advantage is that they can produce a greater improvement in the skin.

Various types of chemical peels exist, each suited to different skin problems and types. Chemical peels are classified as superficial, medium, and deep according to the strength of the formulation and the depth to which they penetrate.

Chemical peels can be used to replace part or all of the top layers of skin. The important factors deciding which chemical peel is perfect for you are; the extent of the skin problem (such as aging or sun-damage), the skin type or color, the amount of improvement you desire, and the length of recovery downtime you are willing to accept.

Parts of the body other than the face can be peeled also. For example, you can have chemical peels on the chest and back for acne, or on the neck and décolletage to help reduce sun damage.

Important note: Deep peeling too frequently can seriously damage the skin. The outermost layer of skin (the stratum corneum) is not a mat of useless, dead cells but a vital protective barrier. It keeps out pollution, conserves moisture, acts as our skin's own natural sunscreen and keeps acne bacteria at bay.

A chemical peel may be beneficial once a month, but if people have these treatments weekly or even more frequently, they will interfere with the skin's protective barrier. This can lead to chronic levels of inflammation, thread veins and blotchy discoloration. Avoid peels altogether if you have certain skin conditions such as acne, broken capillaries or rosacea.

SKIN TYPES AND COLORS

The darker the skin type, the more unwanted side-effects that may arise following peeling treatments. These may include pigmentation problems such as 'post-inflammatory hyperpigmentation', in which the treated skin may become darker than the untreated skin. As a result, deeper peels in darker skin types should be approached cautiously. Frequently it is more appropriate to have a series of superficial peels instead of one deep peel.

The extent of skin damage to aging and exposure will also affect which peel to use. Superficial peels may be all that is needed for younger patients with less sun-damage and pigmentation and fewer wrinkles.

SUPERFICIAL CHEMICAL PEELS

Alpha-hydroxy acid (AHA) peels
Alpha-hydroxy acid peels include glycolic and lactic acid peels. Glycolic acid is derived from sugar cane, and lactic acid occurs naturally in the human body. These peels can be performed at various concentrations to vary the depth of the treatment. Their main role is to remove the top layers of the skin and induce new collagen formation.

Find the instructions for a home-made AHA peels in our 'recipes' section (page 250).

Beta-hydroxy acid (BHA) peels
Salicylic acid is main ingredient found in BHA peels. These formulations are generally used on oilier skins or acne prone skins, as they are oil soluble and penetrate deeper in this type of skin environment.

Beta-hydroxy acids generally have larger molecules than alpha-hydroxy acids and therefore they may not penetrate as deeply in a normal (non-oily) skin environment. Find the instructions for a home-made BHA peel in our 'recipes' section (page 250).

Combination peels

Some peels may contain combinations, for example a mingling of AHAs and BHAs as well as some mechanical exfoliants such as sugar or salt.

Retinoic acid peels

Retinoic acid is the ingredient found in popular skin-care products such as Retin-A or Stieva-A® (tretinoin), although in much less concentrations that in retinoic acid peels.

Retinoic acid helps to increase the cell turnover rate of the skin and make it behave more like a 'younger skin'. It can also help to reduce DNA mutations caused by UV exposure—i.e. the precursors to skin cancers.

Comparison between retinol and retinoic acid:

There is a distinct difference between the actions of retinol, also known as retinyl palmitate or vitamin A, and those of retinoic acid (used in products such as Retin-A and Renova®).

Retinoic acid's proven effects include reducing skin oil, wrinkles and acne. Potential side effects include irritation and redness, and very dry skin. Furthermore it increases production of the scar-forming growth factor (TGF beta 1).

Retinol improves skin moisturization by increasing skin oil, reduces collagen and elastin breakdown, and has very modest wrinkle reducing actions. Its potential unwanted side effects are minimal, but in younger people it can cause breakouts in acne prone skin. It has been an ingredient in skin products for the last 60 years. Some cosmetic facial products that are advertised to contain retinol have only 0.001% retinol—a biologically insignificant amount that has no effect.

Retinol helps to reduce wrinkles mainly by reducing collagen and elastin degradation. A balance of biosynthesis (production of new skin cells) and degradation (breakdown of old skin cells) is essential for healthy skin. However, as we age the balance shifts towards excessive breakdown. Retinol helps block the action of a protein complex called AP-1 which produces the enzymes that break apart and degrade collagen and elastin, the major structural materials in our skin. Thus it retains a balance between healthy and dying skin cells.

Retinol can cause increased acne in persons aged from 18 to 25. Contradictorily, retinol creams can often prevent severe chronic cystic acne in some people between 25 and 40.

When using retinol creams it is best to start with a small amount and build up to larger doses.

Jessner's peel

Jessner's peel is a combination peel of salicylic acid, resorcinol, and lactic acid. Resorcinol is a derivative of phenol (a very deep peeling agent) and is efficacious for resurfacing the skin. The depth of the Jessner's peel is determined by the number of layers of the formulation placed on the skin, but it is usually used as a superficial peel. The skin turns white for a short time after treatment.

Trichloroacetic acid (TCA) chemical peel 10-20%

Performed at lower concentrations, TCA peels provide superficial resurfacing of the skin to improve skin texture, wrinkles, and pigmentation.

MEDIUM DEPTH CHEMICAL PEELS

Trichloroacetic acid (TCA) 35%

At these higher concentrations, TCA peels can help improve skin texture, wrinkles and pigmentation. This is a cost-effective alternative to laser resurfacing.

DEEP CHEMICAL PEELS

Deep peeling involves the use of either trichloracetic acid in concentrations above 50% or formulations containing phenol.

Phenol 88%

One of the strongest peeling agents available for severe wrinkling and sun-damaged skin, phenol 88% can be cardiotoxic (people have died having this peel!) and treatment usually needs to be performed while the patient is under a general anesthetic. There is significant whitening (and sometimes over-whitening) of the skin after this peel.

Baker-Gordon phenol peel

Like the phenol 88% peel, the Baker-Gordon phenol peel is one of the strongest peeling treatments available for heavily damaged skin. It can also have dangerous side effects such as cardiotoxicity, usually requires the administration of a general anesthetic and dramatically whitens the skin.

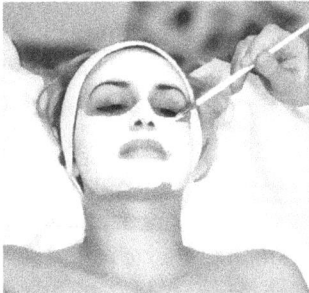

CHOOSING THE RIGHT PEEL

Different skin problems respond to particular peels.

Acne:

Acne responds well to Jessner's peel and BHA peel, both of which contain salicylic acid. These peels are very oil-soluble and are thus able to penetrate deeper into pores to remove oil and sebum. Salicylic acid is also anti-inflammatory.

Large pores, skin texture and dryness.

Both alpha-hydroxy acid and beta-hydroxy acid peels help exfoliate the skin, which can improve all the above conditions. Additionally, serums and moisturizers are more readily absorbed into skin that is not clogged by dead cells, oil and grime.

Discoloration and sun damage:

TCA peels, alpha-hydroxy acid peels, and Jessner's peels are suited to pigmentation problems and sun-damage.

Wrinkles:

Wrinkles can be best treated with TCA peels, or any medium to deep chemical peel. These peels can be a cost-effective alternative to laser resurfacing.

BEFORE AND AFTER A PEEL

Beginning at least two weeks before the peel, the skin should be prepared by applying skin care products containing retinoic acid, as well as topical lightening agents such as hydroquinone, tretinoin, kojic acid or arbutin. This will help with uniform penetration of the peel formula and also speed up the healing process afterwards. Additionally it will reduce post-peel complications such as post-inflammatory hyperpigmentation (dark patches). This skin priming regime is especially important before medium peels or deep peels, and for people with darker skin.

To prevent or ameliorate any pigmentation problems following the peel, it is recommended that patients continue the regime for two weeks afterwards.

The use of alpha-hydroxy acid (AHA) cleansers or exfoliants in the weeks prior to chemical peeling can also help the peeling formula penetrate more evenly, but they do not reduce the risk of post-inflammatory hyperpigmentation.

It is essential to avoid sun exposure as much as possible both before and after a peel. UV rays can cause pigmentation problems, especially in freshly peeled skin.

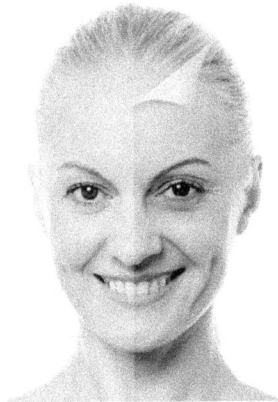

SKIN THERAPY:
DERMABRASION AND MICRODERMABRASION

Dermabrasion and microdermabrasion are terms that refer to the abrasive removal of layers of skin, usually on the face. They are mechanical peels, as distinct from chemical peels. After these procedures, the skin that grows back is generally smoother and fresher.

DERMABRASION VS MICRODERMABRASION

Dermabrasion removes the upper layers of skin right down to the deeper collagen layer. There are very few doctors who still perform dermabrasion. It has largely been replaced all over the world by newer and somewhat simpler technologies including lasers such as the CO2 or Erbium:YAG laser. Laser therapies have the advantage of causing little to no bleeding and are usually less dependent on a skilled operator than dermabrasion.

Dermabrasion should not be confused with microdermabrasion which is a newer and non-surgical cosmetic procedure performed by non-medical staff, nurses, estheticians, medical assistants, or even untrained individuals in a home setting.

Microdermabrasion is a lighter, shallower peel that requires no anesthesia. With microdermabrasion there is less recovery 'downtime' than with dermabrasion. Afterwards the skin pinkish-red, but this blushing fades within 24 hours. Microdermabrasion is useful for people who cannot take time off work to allow the healing process to take place.

Which procedure is best for you?
Consult your esthetician or doctor to find out which procedure would work best for the look you would like to achieve.

①DERMABRASION

Dermabrasion, also called dermaplaning, is a mechanical method of skin peeling. It is a surgical, invasive procedure that usually requires a local anesthetic and is performed in a medical clinic by a dermatologist or cosmetic surgeon trained in this particular technique. Dermabrasion was practiced for many years before the advent of lasers. This procedure is best suited to people with fair skin. For people with darker skin, dermabrasion can result in scarring or discoloration.[47]

Purpose: Its aim is to smooth the skin and help diminish the appearance of deep scars caused by accidents, surgery or disease, pigmentation, pock marks, wrinkles and other skin imperfections. Some patients choose to have their whole face treated with dermabrasion to smooth out acne scarring. The area around the mouth can also be treated, to diminish fine or deep wrinkles. Dermabrasion can improve the appearance of uneven skin tone, sun damage, tattoos, age spots and stretch marks. It is not effective in treating congenital skin defects, most moles, pigmented birthmarks, or scars caused by burns.

How it's done: Dermabrasion involves the controlled, deep abrasion (wearing away) of the upper to mid layers of the skin with any of a variety of strong, abrasive devices such as:
* a rapidly rotating wire brush,
* a rapidly rotating diamond wheel with abrasive edges (called a burr or fraise)
* sterilized sandpaper

After the procedure the skin can be very red and raw-looking. Depending on the level of skin removal, it takes an average of 7–30 days for the skin to fully heal.

Possible risks and complications: Since the procedure removes the top layer and often the deeper layers of the epidermis, extending into the lowest layer of the dermis, there is always a certain amount of bleeding. Dermabrasion carries risks of scarring, skin discoloration, infections, and facial herpes virus (cold sore) reactivation.

---

47   *Dermabrasion. From Wikipedia, the free encyclopedia. Article retrieved November 2014.*

MICRODERMABRASION

Microdermabrasion is a process that deeply exfoliates the skin. The whirling tip of a diamond coated device, called a 'head' or 'wand', comes into contact with the skin and gently abrades the top layer, removing the most superficial cells, which are then vacuumed away.

It can be used to help treat various skin conditions such as:
- acne
- minor acne scarring
- very shallow wrinkles
- uneven skin texture
- comedones (blackheads and whiteheads)
- dull or rough skin
- age spots and other superficial pigmentation
- enlarged pores
- uneven skin tone

Prior to a microdermabrasion session, your face is thoroughly cleansed. The microdermabrasion head is then systematically passed over the treatment area several times. Healing, moisturizing or nourishing creams or serums are applied to the treatment area after the procedure has been completed. The treatment takes around 60 minutes. Usually a few sessions are required for optimal results. The number and frequency of microdermabrasion sessions depends on the patient's skin type and requirements.

Microdermabrasion has three simultaneous actions: exfoliation, vacuum suction (to remove dulling dead skin cells, unblock pores and increase blood circulation) and lymphatic drainage.

This is a non-invasive and relatively comfortable skin treatment. Most people feel very little to no pain during the session. The sensation when having a microdermabrasion treatment can be compared to that of an exfoliating scrub combined with a light facial massage.

Microdermabrasion is a safe and effective procedure. There are very few risks. Patients may experience some transient redness of the treated areas, minor skin flaking and in some cases a mild breakout of pimples. When the after-effects settle down, the skin feels soft and smooth.

Microdermabrasion works on all skin types and colors. It makes subtle improvements, causing no skin color change or scarring. However it is not effective for deeper problems such as scars, stretch marks, wrinkles, or deep acne scars.

This technique is most commonly used on the face, but it can be used on the neck, back, hands, shoulders, chest, upper arms and buttocks.

⊛ SKIN THERAPY: LASER SKIN THERAPIES

Non-surgical skin-tightening procedures such as laser therapies deliver heat into the epidermal and dermal layers of the skin. This creates controlled injury, which encourages the body to produce more collagen in the treated area. The body's natural healing process creates new, healthy tissue to replace the affected areas, resulting in younger-looking skin. Patients may need more than one session.

Over time, the increased collagen produced by laser treatments plumps and thickens the skin, reducing the appearance of fine to moderate lines and wrinkles, acne scarring and numerous other skin problems. There is improvement in skin tone, texture, and tightness. Laser energy may also contract existing collagen fibers to produce an immediate effect. It is, however, not very effective on very deep lines such as nasolabial folds.

There are numerous types of medical lasers, each emitting a certain wavelength that has a different effect on skin. Each laser wavelength is attracted to a particular substance in the tissue. This means that a particular laser wavelength is able to aim at a particular skin problem, depending on what it is attracted to. Some wavelengths will be attracted to melanin (pigment), others to hemoglobin (blood), and others are attracted to the water in the skin. Each wavelength will also penetrate to a different depth.

Both ablative (tissue-destroying) and non-ablative laser technologies can be used on practically any area of the body – limbs, face, neck and torso.

One of the benefits of laser treatment is its specificity. Lasers are able to selectively treat very small areas with minimal or no disruption to the surrounding skin.

The difference between laser and Intense Pulsed Light (IPL)

Lasers have specific wavelengths to focus on specific problems. In contrast, IPL emits a wide spectrum of light with multiple wavelengths. IPL targets several problems simultaneously, and not as selectively as laser. See our section on Intense Pulsed Light (page 217).

Issues that benefit from laser skin therapies include:

- Discolored skin, including melasma, excess pigmentation (brown spots), brown birthmarks, red colored birthmarks (port wine stain) and more
- vascular conditions such as spider veins and superficial, visible, broken capillaries (often associated with conditions such as rosacea)
- facial redness / rosacea
- unwanted tattoo removal
- laser hair removal
- fine or moderate lines and wrinkles such as crow's feet
- skin texture/textural irregularities
- skin laxity
- decreased collagen
- scarring, including indented acne scarring and raised scars—usually keloid or hypertrophic scars
- active acne
- fatty pockets and lumps (another alternative is radiowave surgery)
- stretch marks

TYPES OF LASERS

The many different laser treatments available are usually cataloged according to injury pattern, the depth to which they penetrate the skin, and whether they destroy (ablate) or simply heat the tissue.

The wavelength of the laser decrees how deeply it penetrates the skin. Ablative resurfacing reaches both surface and deeper tissue, resulting in longer post-treatment healing time than non-ablative resurfacing requires. Redness and swelling from ablative procedures may last up to two weeks. The greater the skin injury during treatment, the better the result; however this also means a longer recovery time and a higher risk of unwanted side-effects.

- *Continuous ablative lasers* — the most effective, with correspondingly longer recovery times.
- *Fractional ablative lasers* — a slightly milder effect than continuous ablative, with slightly less recovery time needed.
- *Non-ablative lasers* — a milder effect.
- *Fractional non- ablative lasers* — the most gentle.

Ablative Lasers
* Continuous wave ablative lasers
These lasers vaporize and destroy the affected tissue, which the body then replaces with new, healthy tissue. Continuous ablative laser affects 100% of the skin in the area to be treated. The procedure may need a combination of topical and systemic painkillers and sedation.

Recovery requires a week at home out of the sun keeping the raw skin moist, and it may be red for a few weeks after that. Only one session is needed.

Continuous ablative procedures may result in unwanted side effects such as scarring, redness, changes in pigmentation or infections. This sort of risk is decreased by using fractional ablative lasers instead.

* Fractional ablative lasers

Fractional lasers penetrate the skin in a pattern of tiny columns, leaving surrounding tissue unaffected. This treatment affects surface and deeper tissue, resulting in 'down-time' that is less than continuous ablative treatment but longer than fractional non-ablative treatment. Post-procedural redness and swelling may last up to two weeks. With one to two treatments patients will achieve results such as more even skin time and texture, often with an added bonus of some skin tightening.

Fractional ablative laser treatment can give consistent, long-term results. Brand names of fractional ablative lasers include Fraxel Repair® and Pearl Fractional®.

Non-ablative Lasers

* Continuous wave non-ablative lasers

Continuous wave lasers treat the whole area of skin. Non-ablative lasers heat and coagulate the tissue to stimulate collagen production, but leave it intact. Non-ablative laser treatment requires only a topical anesthetic.

The patient's skin will be red for up to a week, and there may be mild swelling and peeling.

Best results will probably need several sessions a few weeks apart. In a best-case scenario, an immediate improvement can be seen, with continued improvements for the next two to three months.

Some brand names of non-ablative laser include Fraxel Restore® and Laser Genesis®.

* Fractional non-ablative lasers

This is a simple treatment that delivers excellent aesthetic results with minimal redness or swelling.

Unlike ablative lasers, which remove the top layer of skin and part of the sub-layer, non-ablative lasers keep the outer layer of skin in place, for faster healing and recovery. As stated earlier, fractional lasers also penetrate the skin in a pattern of tiny columns, leaving surrounding tissue unaffected. Non-ablative procedures involve minimal to no downtime, but they require a course of several treatments.

Advantages include:
- Good results with minimal recovery time
- Little to no pain during the procedure
- Reduced redness or swelling
- Suits most skin types

* Combination ablative and non-ablative laser
The combination of ablative and non-ablative fractional lasers creates a treatment that takes advantage of the best of both technologies. This approach can provide dramatic yet natural-looking results by improving fine lines and wrinkles and treating unwanted pigmentation with as little as three days of recovery.

Pulsed Dye Lasers
Pulsed dye lasers (PDL) convey a powerful surge of light into carefully targeted areas of the skin. Your practitioner will adjust the laser's settings so that the light will be absorbed by particular blood vessels or melanin pigmented areas in your skin, depending on which condition you are being treated for.

Pulsed dye lasers can treat the following skin issues:
- redness of the face and neck
- red, broken blood vessels showing under the skin
- rosacea
- spider veins
- freckles
- age spots
- mild scars and red stretch marks
- warts
- early signs of sun-damage
- port wine stains

Depending on the skin disorder for which you are being treated, you may need more than one treatment session. Brand names of Pulsed Dye Lasers include Vbeam Perfecta® and Flashlamp Pulsed Dye Laser.

Infrared Lasers

Infrared skin therapy is also known as 'red light therapy' or 'photorejuvenation'. It is non-surgical. The function and purpose of infrared skin treatment is to reduce the appearance of wrinkles, remodel skin, improve acne and acne scars, and treat sebaceous hyperplasia.

A study published in August 2006 concluded that: '... infrared radiation may have beneficial effects on skin texture and wrinkles by increasing collagen and elastin contents from the stimulated fibroblasts. Therefore, skin treatment with infrared radiation may be an effective and safe non-ablative remodeling method, and may also be useful in the treatment of photo-aged skin.'[48]

There is a variety of infrared systems on the market, including (though not limited to) the following brand names: CoolTouch®, SmoothBeam®, Erbium Glass laser, Titan® and Sciton SkinTyte®. The main action of the red light waves is that they bypass the epidermis (the skin's top layer) and become absorbed throughout the dermis. This brings about dermal heating. Dermal heating with infrared energy creates both immediate and long-term benefits.

Skin tightening and wrinkle/scar reduction

The immediate benefit of infrared laser treatment is heat-induced collagen shrinkage, which leads to mild skin tightening and a decrease in wrinkles. On average, wrinkle improvements are moderate: small and medium wrinkles and acne scars (especially pitted ones) often noticeably improve. Deep wrinkles, especially those due to facial movement, are less likely to improve.

Skin remodeling

More significantly, the longer-term benefit of infrared laser treatment is skin remodeling (new collagen growth in the deeper

---

48   *Effects of Infrared Radiation on Skin Photo-Aging and Pigmentation. Ju Hee Lee, Mi Ryung Roh, and Kwang Hoon Lee, Yonsei Medical Journal.*

skin layers), which continues unabated for up to six months after the initial treatment. This is thought to produce a lasting improvement in wrinkles and some skin tightening, although individual outcomes vary.

Acne improvement

Some infrared systems, such as CoolTouch® and SmoothBeam®, seem to have a beneficial effect on acne. Apparently the treatment decreases the size and activity of sebaceous glands, reducing the production of skin oil, one of the factors causing acne.

TYPES OF LASERS USED FOR 'FACELIFTS'

Subdermal Laser Threading

With this technique, the practitioner places an ultra-thin laser fiber just below the surface of the skin. Laser energy passes through the fiber. It heats up the skin's natural collagen and elastin fibers, causing them to contract and tighten the skin, while permanently melting small fatty deposits.

The patient undergoes a light sedation and the neck is numbed with a local anesthetic. A tiny incision is made in the corner of the neck and under the chin. The laser fiber is passed under the skin.

Results continue to appear over the following 6—9 weeks with significant improvement in the overall skin quality without the need for surgical skin removal.

This procedure takes about one hour. It is considered a safe procedure with minimum side effects. After the treatment, patients can get back to their routine activities within a day or two.

There will be swelling in the treated area for 3—7 days with minimal bruising. Very rarely, a patient may develop a blister in the area, but only if too much laser heat has been applied. Patients need to wear a close-fitting elastic garment for three days full time, and then for another seven days part time.

Subdermal laser threading treatment can also be carried out on areas of the face, stomach, cheeks and upper arms.

TYPES OF LASERS USED TO TIGHTEN SKIN

Infrared lasers

Infrared lasers (page 211) are used to shrink and tighten collagen while stimulating new collagen production for firmer, smoother skin. This is a non-surgical option for sagging skin, especially if is carried out the first sign of drooping. Advanced laxity doesn't respond well to infrared laser treatment. Of course this treatment is no substitute for a face-lift, and any tightening of the skin happen gradually. Full results can take as long as six months to be visible.

Infrared laser requires 3–4 treatments for best results. Trade names include Titan®.

TYPES OF LASERS USED FOR REMOVING FATTY POCKETS

Liposuction Lasers

Smartlipo® (also referred to as SmartLipo, Smart Lipo, Smart Liposuction, and Laser Liposuction) uses laser energy to liquefy fat before it is removed via a small tube called a cannula.

Learn more in the section on laser liposuction under 'Liposuction' (page 178).

TYPES OF LASERS USED FOR SKIN RESURFACING

Carbon dioxide (CO2) Laser

The carbon dioxide laser was invented in 1964 and estheticians still find it one of the most useful. Carbon dioxide lasers are the highest-powered ablative lasers that are currently available. They vaporize the top layers of the skin (epidermis) and cause it to regenerate with fewer wrinkles and improved tightness. They can treat a variety of skin issues including wrinkles, scars, warts and enlarged oil glands on the nose.

CO2 lasers target the deep layer (dermis) in which lie collagen and other elements that make for high quality skin. The laser heats this layer to an optimum temperature which stimulates it, thus promoting remodeling of the dermis to produce fresh, healthy skin.

The skin can take one to two weeks to heal and can be red for one to two months afterwards. Risks of scarring, skin discoloration, and uneven texture must be weighed against the intended outcome, although these side effects are rare when the doctor is experienced with this kind of procedure.

Although the CO2 laser can create more lasting and noticeable results than any other laser, it is also associated with the most risk and potential skin damage.

Carbon dioxide lasers may be continuous ablative or fractional ablative. With fractional carbon dioxide lasers, small columns of laser are fired into the skin, while parts of the skin in between these columns are left untreated. This helps to reduce the risk and allows for safer treatment than traditional (continuous) carbon dioxide lasers.

Trade names of CO2 lasers include Feather Touch® and Ultra Pulse®.

Erbium: YAG Laser

This ablative laser is far less invasive than the CO2 laser and is considered effective for minor or superficial wrinkling. However, if the intensity of the machine's energy emissions is increased, deeper wrinkling can also be treated.

Erbium fractional laser skin resurfacing is designed to remove surface-level and moderately deep lines and wrinkles on the face, hands, neck, or chest. One of the benefits of erbium laser resurfacing is minimal burning of surrounding tissue.

The erbium laser causes fewer side effects than the CO2 laser — such as swelling, bruising, and redness — so that recovery time should be faster than with CO2 laser resurfacing. In some cases, recovery may only take one week. Erbium laser resurfacing is more suitable for people with a darker skin tone.

Variable Pulse YAG Laser

Another skin resurfacing option is the Variable Pulse YAG Laser, which alternates light frequency with pulses that heat the skin and cause ablation. This resurfaces the skin almost as effectively as CO2, but with fewer side effects.

Combination of CO2 and Erbium: YAG laser

In this treatment, the erbium laser is first used to remove the epidermis, followed by use of the CO2 laser to achieve contraction of underlying collagen. This produces the collagen-tightening benefits of CO2 therapy but with minimal damage to surrounding tissues.

Fractional Photothermolysis Laser

This procedure delivers hundreds to thousands of microscopic, pixelated thermal (heat) injuries to skin, with the goal being to stimulate collagen production for smoother, firmer skin. The pinpoint injuries this light treatment causes do not affect surrounding skin, so you can get impressive results with less down time and less risky side effects (when compared to CO2 laser resurfacing). Fractional Photothermolysis Laser treatments can be of benefit to people with superficial acne scarring.

There is generally very little downtime associated with fractional resurfacing. Patients may notice lingering redness or brown spots for a month or so afterward, but these vanish in time. For best results, a series of 2–4 treatments is recommended.

Trade names include Affirm®, Fraxel®, Active-Fx® and Lux 1540.

Long-Pulsed YAG Laser

This non-ablative laser is often used to treat wrinkles and reduce the appearance of acne scars. As with any non-ablative laser resurfacing, it takes several treatments to achieve very subtle results. Treatment needs to be repeated every year or two to maintain the results and help discourage further sagging. Long-Pulsed YAG Lasers can also be used for hair removal and treating surface capillaries.

Trade names include CoolTouch® and Lyra®.

Q-Switched Ruby Laser

This laser is minimally ablative and is primarily used to selectively remove skin pigment, such as freckling, sun-damage spots, and actinic keratosis without damaging the surrounding tissue. It is also useful for removing birthmarks. It usually takes several treatments to achieve the desired results. One of the most common uses for the Q-Switched Ruby laser is cosmetic tattoo removal.

Pulsed Dye Laser (See page 210)

This non-ablative laser removes surface capillaries on the face, port wine marks, thick or raised scars, and hemangiomas (red dots on the surface of skin). It doesn't cause skin damage, but it almost always causes temporary bruising. Several treatments may be required.

Trade names include Candela® and VBeam®.

Long-Pulsed Alexandrite Laser

This non-ablative laser is another option for hair removal and removing surfaced capillaries and leg veins. This machine quickly covers large areas of skin.

Trade names include GentleLASE® and Cool Pulse®.

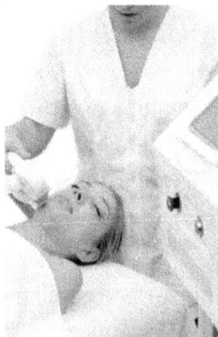

SKIN THERAPY: INTENSE PULSED LIGHT (IPL)

Intense Pulsed Light (IPL) is a non-surgical skin tightening procedure. It is distinct from laser therapy. The two techniques are often confused. IPL machines are not lasers, despite the fact that, like lasers, they work by emitting light to cause selective thermal damaging of the target area. The primary difference is that laser treatment uses laser-generated coherent and monochromatic light (light of a single color). IPL emits incoherent, polychromatic (many-colored) light.

IPL uses bursts of intense light energy to heat the epidermis and dermis. Different programs are entered into the machine to allow targeting of different problems. A specific device is attached to the machine for hair removal treatments.

Skin Discoloration

IPL is used for the improvement of skin tone and surface imperfections associated with aging and sun damage, such as discoloration and superficial brown spots. It may not, however, have much effect on wrinkles. Broken capillaries and general redness may also be treated.

IPL is also useful in the treatment of rosacea and – in combination with ALA (Alpha Lipoic Acid) cream – in managing acne.

Patients may experience a mild stinging sensation as a pulse of light is delivered. After treatment, the skin may be red for a few hours. Any brown spots of skin discoloration will start to darken, and after one to two weeks these spots will flake off in tiny scales before fading. Treatment time is less than one hour.

Two to five treatments are usually recommended, at four-week intervals, with maintenance treatments a few times a year. The improvement is gradual, and it may take a few sessions before patients notice the difference.

Skin Texture

With repeated treatments, IPL can provide collagen stimulation and therefore some tissue remodeling over time, which means skin may also look younger. The increased collagen thickens and plumps up the skin, reducing the appearance of acne scarring, fine lines and stretch marks, and improving skin texture and elasticity.

A series of three to six treatments is usually recommended, with maintenance treatments several times a year. The improvement is gradual, and you may have a few sessions before you notice the difference.

This procedure has no downtime, though patients may notice minor swelling, tenderness, and in rare cases some bruising, which fades within days.

Hair Removal

Intense Pulsed Light devices can also be used for hair removal, and gets result that are as good as most lasers. Before treatment, the skin must be shaved. Treatment can be painful; it feels like being flicked with a stretched elastic band. Cold tips on the IPL device reduce pain and help to protect the upper layers of skin from burning.

The target for laser hair removal is the pigment in the relatively large hair bulbs that lie in the deep layers of the skin. A number of different lasers and IPL devices can be used to target the pigmented hair bulb as long as they penetrate deeply enough. Usually it is dark thick hair that responds best; IPL may have little or no effect on blond or red hair.

Trade names

There are many names used for intense pulsed light treatments. Some trade names of IPL machines include Limelight® by Cutera, FotoFacial®, PhotoFacial®, PhotoDerm®, EpiLight®, MultiLight®, PlasmaLight®, Lumenis,® Quantum®, and Palomar Starlux®.

SKIN THERAPY: LED LIGHT THERAPY

LED light therapy uses narrow band light emitting diodes (LEDs) to target skin cells and make improvements in a wide range of skin issues.

The treatment is pain free and non-invasive. LED is used to treat acne, fine lines and wrinkles, pigmentation, acne scarring and rosacea. It can also soothe the skin and reduce redness and inflammation. The skin's collagen production is increased by this treatment. Enhanced collagen production decreases wrinkles and improves the overall texture of the skin, resulting in a more youthful appearance and texture.

LED light therapy machines use light in a variety colors, each of which is aimed at different skin problems. Your esthetician will discuss your concerns with you and match the settings to your particular needs.

Blue light therapy can sterilize. It is used to eradicate bacteria, and it is very useful for treating acne and oily/acne prone skin.

Red light therapy calms and heals the skin, promoting collagen production and encouraging cell renewal. This light is used to reduce wrinkles as well as to hydrate and tighten the skin.

Trade names include Omnilux®.

SKIN THERAPY: LOW LEVEL LASER THERAPY

Low Level Laser Therapy (LLLT) is also known as Cold Laser Therapy, Soft Laser Therapy, Red Light Laser, light-emitting diode phototherapy, Bio-Modulation, Photo Biostimulation and LED photo therapy.

This non-surgical technique uses red and infrared light which is non-thermal, and therefore does not burn or heat. It is an excellent solution for people who have sustained any type of wound, whether surgical or accidental. This technology is also used to treat numerous skin conditions that need stimulation for healing, relief of pain and inflammation, and restoration of function.

Wound Healing, Skin Laxity, Pigmentation and More

LLLT is designed to speed up the wound healing process by stimulating the circulation of the blood in the smallest blood vessels, thus delivering more oxygen and nutrients to the target area via a process so called photo biostimulation.

By accelerating the body's natural healing process, LLLT can have a beneficial effect on bruises, infections, bed sores, wound ulceration, chronic wounds and surgical wounds. It is used to treat acne, skin laxity, musculoskeletal problems pigmentation problems and more. LLLT causes an increase in the development of the skin's collagen and it has also been shown to be useful in pain management. Results, however, may vary from patient to patient.

'The skin responds well to red and near-infrared wavelengths. Stem cells can be activated, allowing increased tissue repair and healing. In dermatology, Low Level Laser Therapy has beneficial effects on wrinkles, acne scars, hypertrophic scars, and healing of burns. Low Level Laser Therapy can reduce UV damage. In pigmentary disorders such as vitiligo, Low Level Laser Therapy can increase or decrease pigmentation.

'Inflammatory diseases such as psoriasis and acne can also be managed. The noninvasive nature and almost complete absence of side effects encourage further testing in dermatology.'[49]

Low Level Laser Therapy devices have been used around the globe for more than 30 years. The technology has been proven safe in more than 3000 international studies. Currently, the FDA (in the USA) has cleared more than 25 different LLLT devices for a range of treatments for a huge variety of problems.

It is important that patients undergo a full series of treatment sessions to obtain the best results.

---

49   *Semin Cutan Med Surg 32:41-52 © 2013 Frontline Medical Communications.*

Benefits of Low Level Laser Therapy for the skin include:

- A smoother appearance for the skin
- Reduction of puffy eyes and dark circles
- Reduction of pore sizes
- Refining of skin texture
- Improvement of skin tone
- Boosting of collagen production
- Increase in circulation
- Promotion of lymphatic drainage
- Activation of cell metabolic function
- Stimulation of new cell formation and growth
- Renewed and rejuvenated skin
- Improvement in stretch marks, burns and scars
- Improvement of pigmentation marks

Other benefits of Low Level Laser Therapy include:

- Cervical (neck pain) healing
- Lumbar (low back pain) healing
- Relief of wrist pain and injuries (carpal tunnel)
- Relief of elbow and joint pain and injuries
- Lower extremities pain relief
- Foot and ankle pain relief
- Joint pain and knee injury relief
- Accelerated recovery after surgery

There are two basic styles for treatment using cold lasers; pinpoint treatments (laserpuncture) and broad therapy. Each treatment style has a different goal and different equipment requirements.

Some brand names of Low Level Laser Therapy include RENEW ME® Laser Lift, TerraQuant TQ Solo®, Erchonia PL5000, Theralase®, Medx Console®, DJO Vectra Genesis®, Apollo® and K-laser®.

SKIN THERAPY:
MICROCURRENT COSMETIC REJUVENATION

Microcurrent Cosmetic Rejuvenation (also known as electrotherapy) is a non-surgical facial sculpting treatment for the skin. This technique can sculpt, lift and tighten the skin on the face or any part of the body. It can rejuvenate the skin by tightening sagging jowls and softening wrinkles around the eyes, on the brow and around the mouth and cheeks. It can also improve the appearance of acne scarring, rosacea, cellulite and stretch marks.

Microcurrent treatment involves passing a very small direct electrical current (micro-ampere current) through muscle tissue. This stimulates healthy collagen remodeling inside the skin.

This treatment offers advantages for clients who want quick results without the risk of surgery. There is little, if any, discomfort during the treatment. Patients may see some minor improvements after 3—4 treatments, and good results after 15—20 treatments.

Microcurrent cosmetic rejuvenation works by 'retraining' the muscle tissue. It is recommended that patients attend a series of treatment sessions over several weeks, for best results. Practitioners of this method say that if the entire series of treatments is completed and the patient attends regular maintenance sessions, the improvement should last 3—4 years.

Other skin resurfacing procedures stimulate collagen by injuring the deeper layers of the skin (dermis). Microcurrent does not work by injuring; nor does it require a period of healing to produce results.

Besides the face and neck, microcurrent cosmetic rejuvenation can also treat the stomach, legs, hands, back, arms, and buttocks.

Microcurrent therapy may help to:

- Plump upper lip lines
- Lift droopy mouth corners
- Lift a drooping nose
- Erase or smooth dark circles and bags under the eyes
- Tighten sagging skin
- Improve the appearance of jowls and pouches
- Remove droopy fat or fluid from beneath the chin
- Lift sagging upper eyelids
- Lift and define cheek bones
- Tighten 'turkey neck' throat
- Reduce the appearance of wrinkles on the brow, around the eyes and elsewhere
- Lift the eyebrows

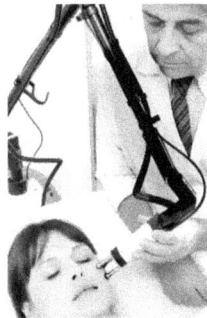

SKIN THERAPY: PHOTODYNAMIC THERAPY

Photodynamic therapy (PDT), sometimes called photochemotherapy, is a form of phototherapy using nontoxic light-sensitive compounds which, when exposed to light, become toxic to targeted malignant and other diseased skin cells. PDT has proven ability to kill bacteria, fungi and viruses.

It is a non-surgical procedure.

Photodynamic therapy is used to treat acne. It is also used clinically to treat a wide range of medical conditions, including wet age-related macular degeneration and malignant cancers. It is recognised as being both minimally invasive and minimally toxic.

The treatment is effective for some minor skin lesions such as superficial basal cell carcinomas and actinic keratoses (also called solar keratoses). The technique involves gently removing any crust from the lesion and applying a photosensitizing cream. The cream contains an ingredient that is preferentially absorbed by the cancer cells and is sensitive to the special light that is shone onto the treatment area for a few minutes. The light is absorbed by the cancer cells, causing them to be destroyed. This is how PDT selectively destroys the skin cancer whilst preserving the normal surrounding skin.

On some occasions the photodynamic therapy procedure is repeated one week later to increase the cure rate. Photodynamic therapy provides an excellent cosmetic result as it has a lower risk of scarring compared with surgery and has a relatively high success rate, but it can only be used on certain types of skin cancer.

Some brand names of photodynamic therapy devices include: BLU-U® Blue Light Photodynamic Therapy Illuminator.

SKIN THERAPY: PLASMA SKIN REGENERATION

ABOUT PLASMA SKIN REGENERATION

Plasma skin regeneration (PSR), is a non-laser treatment that uses a device to deliver energy in the form of a gas called 'plasma' to rejuvenate and tighten skin, improving facial lines and wrinkles and skin pigmentation associated with sun damage.

Plasma skin regeneration technology uses energy delivered from plasma rather than light or radiofrequency. It delivers millisecond pulses of nitrogen-based plasma to the skin via a handpiece. Within the handpiece an ultra-high-frequency (UHF) generator excites inert nitrogen gas, which is converted into activated ionised gas called plasma. This plasma-containing energy is directed through a quartz nozzle out of the tip of the handpiece and onto the skin. The energy produces a heating action that works at the skin's surface to remove old photodamaged epidermal cells, and below the skin surface or dermis to promote collagen growth.

Plasma skin regeneration devices can be used at varying energy levels to achieve differing results. The amount of energy delivered ranges from 1–4 Joules per pulse. Currently there are three recommended treatment protocols:

- PSR1 – low-energy (1-1.2 Joules) treatments spaced 3 weeks apart
- PSR2 – one high-energy pass (3-4 Joules) performed in a single treatment
- PSR3 – two high-energy passes (3-4 Joules) performed in a single treatment

Although all protocols improve fine lines, tone and texture, and skin pigmentations, it appears that skin/tissue tightening is more pronounced with high-energy treatments.

The low-energy treatments produce results gradually over time and have very little, if any, associated downtime. Most patients can have their first treatment at their first consultation and return to their daily activities directly afterwards.

ISSUES IMPROVED BY PLASMA SKIN REGENERATION

Plasma skin regeneration is best used to treat the early signs of aging such as:

- age spots and skin discoloration (hyperpigmentation)
- slight jowling
- loosening skin
- creasing around the nose and mouth
- wrinkling around the nose and mouth

AN OUTLINE OF THE PSR PROCEDURE

Before treatment takes place, the doctor or esthetician discusses with the patient which areas are to be treated and what the patient's goals are. The doctor may also take some photographs of the proposed treatment areas. For low-energy PSR1 treatment a topical anesthetic cream is applied one hour prior to treatment. For higher energy PSR treatments, a combination of a breathable analgesic and a high-strength topical anesthetic cream are generally used.

During treatment the amount of energy absorbed is affected by how well the skin is hydrated. Dry skin absorbs more energy. For this reason, just before each area receives pulses of plasma energy, the anesthetic cream is wiped dry.

A full-face treatment usually takes less than 15 minutes if performed with PSR1, but treatment with high energy PSR3 takes around 45 minutes because it requires two high energy passes.

Post-treatment and recovery

Low-energy PSR1 treatments may cause mild redness of the skin that lasts 2—3 days. Some flaking of the skin may occur when dead skin is replaced with new skin.

Higher energy plasma skin regeneration treatments will cause mild to moderate redness of the skin in addition to the skin turning brown and shedding or flaking over the next 5—10 days after treatment. To avoid scarring, patients should not pick at or peel their skin.

During the healing phase and for several months after treatment, the treatment area should be shielded from UV rays using a moisturizing sunblock with an SPF of at least 30+. Protective clothing and wide-brimmed hats should also be used.

Usually results are immediate and progressive. Improvement continues for at least a year after treatment.

Potential side effects and complications

Plasma skin regeneration appears to be very well tolerated by most patients, particularly low-energy treatments. Shaving or application of make-up can be done soon after treatment. In most cases, patients can return to work directly after treatments or the following day, depending upon their skin condition and the strength of the plasma energy.

Some of the side effects and complications that may occur, especially after higher energy level treatments include:

- Excessive scaling and peeling of the skin, and some crusting.
- Redness and swelling for up to one week after treatment. This can be ameliorated by applying an ice pack at ten minute intervals for the first 24 hours.
- When patients have received PSR3 with two high energy passes, redness can persist up to 6 to 8 weeks after treatment.
- Temporary hyperpigmentation.

Brand names of plasma skin regeneration include Portrait®.

SKIN THERAPY: PLATELET RICH PLASMA INJECTIONS (PRP INJECTIONS)

Platelet-rich plasma injections (PRP injections) are used in the treatment of musculoskeletal injuries as well as in cosmetic medicine.

Platelet-rich plasma is blood plasma that has been enriched with extra platelets. As a concentrated source of platelets, PRP releases a number of different growth factors and other natural healing cells in the patient's own blood that encourage the healing and regeneration of skin and bone.

Because the patient's own plasma is used, there is no risk of disease transmission, allergy, anaphylaxis or neoplasia.

PRP is suitable for people between the ages of 30 and 80 years.

Platelets are amazing blood cells with many functions. The growth factors they contain can:

- Regenerate and rejuvenate tissue.
- Increase collagen production, leading to increased skin thickness, plumpness and firmness.
- Draft other cells to help with wound healing.
- Encourage the production of molecules that provide structural and biochemical support to the surrounding tissue cells.
- Provide a 'biological glue' for tissue adhesion.
- Improve skin texture and tone.
- Rejuvenate facial skin, including fine wrinkles, in people with mild sun-damage or signs of aging.

PRP is used to treat:

- The area around the eyes where the skin tends to be thin and crêpey, with fine lines (peri-orbital region).
- Acne scarring.
- Cheeks and mid face.
- Thinning skin on the neck.
- The jaw line and chin.
- The area below the cheekbones (sub malar).
- The backs of hands (dorsum).
- The upper part of the torso, comprising neck, shoulders and chest (décolletage).
- The forehead.

Other body areas that can be treated with PRP include knees, elbows, upper arms and 'post-baby' abdomen.

The Procedure:

Patients should be assessed by a medical professional who will examine the skin, recommend an appropriate treatment and discuss it with the patient. This step is important, because skin diseases have to be excluded.

Your clinician will take a photograph of the skin, to aid in monitoring future improvements. You will then have a small amount of blood drawn from your arm via a needle (venapuncture). Your blood will be centrifuged, in the clinic, to separate the plasma, which is then drawn into a syringe.

A topical local anesthesia will be applied to the area to be treated. This makes the procedure relatively pain-free. Next, your clinician will inject the PRP, by inserting multiple tiny punctures into the upper and lower layers of skin (epidermis and dermis).

The procedure usually takes between 45 minutes and one hour in total. PRP facial rejuvenation can be a one-off treatment, but if your lines and wrinkles are persistent, your clinician can perform further microinjections at 6—12 weekly intervals.

SKIN THERAPY: RADIOFREQUENCY SKIN THERAPY

Radiofrequency skin therapy, sometimes known as thermal skin therapy, is used for the non-surgical tightening of slightly loose or sagging skin. It is said to be a good way to rejuvenate the face without the expense and downtime of surgery, though of course the results are not as dramatic as the results of surgery.

This technique is best suited to patients in their mid 30s to 50s of any skin color, who have mild to moderate skin looseness and wrinkling. Radiofrequency is generally employed to treat the forehead, the delicate skin beneath the eyes, the cheeks, the mid-face, the jaw line and the neck. The procedure is frequently used for toning the thin, loose and crepe-like skin often found on the aging face and neck, and under the upper arms.

Radiofrequency is also used for firming abdominal skin on the chest, thighs or breasts, or after surgery or childbirth.

Like ultrasound and infrared treatments, radiofrequency skin therapy is a thermal therapy – that is, it uses heat to achieve results. Radiofrequency skin therapy devices deliver heat deep into the skin, causing collagen fibers to contract and new collagen to form. This tightens lax skin.

After treatment most patients will experience some minor swelling and perhaps some pinkness; side effects which disappear in a few days. Patients can expect to see at least a slight improvement in their skin tightness over time.

One of the major benefits over surgical procedures is that the body generates its own collagen, during and after the treatment for many months to come. This tightens the skin and connective tissue, while increasing blood circulation and assisting with lymphatic drainage.

Radiofrequency skin tightening alone does not lift muscle, unlike a surgical face lift. It neither corrects sun damage nor reduces hollows caused by age-related fat loss. Therefore it is best used in combination with other treatments, such as dermal fillers and laser resurfacing or a chemical peel.

For some people the radiofrequency skin tightening process is uncomfortable, and they may need topical anesthetic. There may be some redness of the skin afterwards, which can be camouflaged with make-up.

The full cosmetic improvement takes a few months to appear, because the skin needs time to produce more collagen. The final effect may last for a few years. Cost depends on the clinic and the amount of coverage (full face, half face etc).

Brands of radiofrequency skin therapy devices include: Accent™ Pellevé™ Thermage® Anti-aging XRF and TriPollar™

SKIN THERAPY:
RADIOFREQUENCY MICRONEEDLING

Radiofrequency microneedling is an excellent treatment for acne and acne scarring. It is also used in facial rejuvenation to tighten and lift skin, and to improve the appearance of wrinkles, large pores, stretch marks and spider veins (telangiectasia). Radiofrequency energy can destroy the causes of acne and acne bacteria.

Fractional radiofrequency microneedling induces selective heating in the deep layers of the dermis, leaving undamaged columns of tissue between the targeted areas. Because it conveys energy deep down into the dermis and does not heat up the epidermis, greater levels of energy can be poured into the target area at the point where the microneedles are inserted. This averts damage to the epidermis, such as burning or hyperpigmentation. It also encourages shortening and tightening of the collagen fibers, and reconstruction of new collagen by the stimulation of fibroblasts.

Radiofrequency microneedling differs from laser treatment in that electroenergy is transformed into thermal energy. The microneedles are insulated except for the final 0.3mm at the end of the needle, from which the radiofrequency energy is emitted. The energy from the needle point is transferred to the tissue, causing coagulation and cell disruption in the surrounding dermis. The energy is only delivered to the dermis, without any heat release into the epidermis.

Before the procedure, a local or topical anesthetic is applied to the area to be treated to make the patient more comfortable. The device is then applied to the skin surface, releasing the needles and delivering radiofrequency energy in short bursts as the device's head is moved across the skin. Immediately afterwards, the treated area will appear red and slightly inflamed. If the patient is uncomfortable, a cool pack, or cold air is applied to the area.

Brands of radiofrequency microneedling devices include: INTRAcel®.

See also the section on 'skin microneedling,' page 238.

SKIN THERAPY:
RADIOWAVE SURGERY FOR SKIN LESIONS

Numerous cosmetic procedures are available to treat warts, moles, skin tags, and other lumps and bumps on the skin. One of the most popular is radiowave surgery, or radiofrequency surgery. A particular band of high frequency radio wavelengths that generate minimal heat can be used for skin surgery. These wavelengths, when channeled through an electrode tip, can cut the skin, simultaneously coagulating the blood to produce a bloodless incision. Surrounding tissues are unaffected.

Compared with the traditional method of removing skin bumps and lumps via surgical incisions, radiowave surgery has many advantages. Although traditional surgery using a scalpel is effective in removing skin imperfections, it can cause scarring, and necessitates a relatively long recovery time that may last for months.

Radiofrequency surgery recovery time is usually between 7 to 10 days. After 10 days, the skin should appear slightly red and will heal completely. This technique leaves little to no scarring and the incisions are bacteria-free. Furthermore, it enhances the skin healing process by causing less pain and swelling.

When used in removing benign skin lesions, radiowave surgery can gradually plane away the lump or bump until the exact skin level is reached. Radiofrequency surgery is used to make incisions on the eyelid in a cosmetic procedure called blepharoplasty.

Dressing is not required after radiofrequency surgery, but the treated skin area is generally covered with a skin-colored medical tape to protect the healing skin from bacteria.

SKIN THERAPY: SKIN LIGHTENING CREAMS

Topical skin lightening agents, also known as skin lightening creams or serums, are used to help reduce skin pigmentation and treat skin discoloration problems.

Generally speaking, lightening agents do not completely remove pigmentation, but they do make it fade significantly. They can be used alone or in conjunction with other therapies, such as laser. In most cases, laser can completely remove pigmentation such as freckles or sunspots. See our section on laser skin therapies (page 206).

Skin lightening creams help to reduce pigmentation by inhibiting the enzymes that produce melanin (skin pigment) and by increasing the turnover of the skin, which flushes out existing pigmentation.

The first defense against skin pigmentation is preventing it from happening or from getting worse. You can help protect your skin from sun damage by applying a good sunscreen every day. Use a topical lightening agent in conjunction with your sunscreen.

Topical lightening agents can treat many types of skin pigmentation, including melasma, chloasma, freckles and sunspots. They are also used to treat post-inflammatory hyperpigmentation (worsening of pigmentation) which may occur after laser skin treatments, chemical or laser peels, or acne treatments.

Topical lightening agents can also be used to prepare the skin for laser treatments. This reduces the risk of post-inflammatory hyperpigmentation, especially for olive to dark skin types. Note that most lightening agents cannot be used during pregnancy or breast-feeding.

The appropriate topical skin lightening agent for each individual depends on-

- their type of pigmentation
- the cause of the pigmentation
- their skin type, e.g. sensitive skin
- their skin color, e.g. pale or dark skin

COMMON ACTIVE AGENTS IN SKIN LIGHTENING CREAMS

Hydroquinone – This chemical compound is the most widely used and efficacious skin lightening agent. It can be used for melasma or chloasma, post-inflammatory hyperpigmentation and other pigmentation disorders. Over the counter, you can buy products with hydroquinone strengths up to 2%. For higher concentrations, you'll need a doctor's prescription. Hydroquinone may be the sole active ingredient in the formulation, or it may be compounded with some of the other agents listed below. Hydroquinone can be somewhat irritating to the skin. It has been known to cause redness or contact dermatitis when used in higher strengths.

Rarely, some people may react to hydroquinone by developing ochronosis in the treated area, which is actually the opposite to the intended effect. Ochronosis is an increase in pigmentation. This rare side effect is generally confined to darker-skinned individuals, and usually only after prolonged use. Alternating the use of hydroquinone with other lightening agents every four months can help to forestall this problem.

Kojic acid – This lightening agent is derived from fungus such as aspergillus and penicillium. It can be used in concentrations between 1% and 4% and can be compounded with other agents. As with hydroquinine, irritation can occur with the use of kojic acid. It is not as effective as hydroquinone, but the advantage is that there is no risk of rebound pigmentation or ochronosis.

Paper mulberry – Paper mulberry extract is isolated from the roots of an ornamental tree, *Broussonetia papyrifera*. A Korean study compared it to kojic acid and hydroquinone, and found that only 0.396% paper mulberry was required to inhibit the enzyme tyrosinase that produces melanin, in comparison to 5.5% hydroquinone and 10% kojic acid. Skin irritation with paper mulberry is less than with other lightening agents such as hydroquinone.

Arbutin – originating from the plant bearberry (Arctostaphylos uva-ursi), arbutin helps to lighten the skin by inhibition of the enzymes that help produce melanin. Like paper mulberry, it is less irritating than kojic acid and hydroquinone.

Niacinamide – Niacinamide is a form of vitamin B3. It inhibits the transfer of the pigment-forming cells, the melanosomes, to the surface of the skin.[50]

Vitamin C – Topical vitamin C (ascorbic acid) also helps interfere with pigment production. An additional benefit of vitamin C is the anti-oxidant effect it bestows, which helps protect skin from environmental damage such as pollution. Vitamin C also stimulates the production of collagen. It can be unstable when it's used in topical products, so either choose a commercial product that's stabilized, or make your own fresh Vitamin C serum at home and use it straight away.

See the recipe for "Vitamin C Serum" on page 273.

Glycolic acid — Glycolic acid is an alpha-hydroxy acid (AHA) that can have a disruptive effect on the top layer of skin, to help exfoliate any pigmented skin cells. By doing so, it speeds skin turnover and

---

50   *Greatens, A; Hakozaki, T; Koshoffer, A; Epstein, H; Schwemberger, S; Babcock, G; Bissett, D; Takiwaki, H; Arase, S; Wickett, RR; Boissy, RE. Effective inhibition of melanosome transfer to keratinocytes by lectins and niacinamide is reversible. Exp. Dermatol 2005, 14, 498–508, doi:10.1111/j.0906-6705.2005.00309.x.*

pigment is lost more rapidly. The glycolic acid in commercial skin-care formulations is usually synthesized in a laboratory. However, glycolic acid can also be obtained from natural sources, such as sugarcane, sugar beets, pineapple, cantaloupe, and unripe grapes.

See "Home-made Skin Care: skin lightening treatments" on page 291.

Retinoids – Retinoids are derived from vitamin A. It is believed that they reduce pigmentation by inhibiting the enzymes causing pigmentation, dispersing pigment granules in the top layer of skin, and accelerating skin turnover to help pigmented skin cells be sloughed more rapidly. It is also this last characteristic that helps retinoids to smooth the skin, soften wrinkles, and reduce active acne. Retinoids can be irritating to the skin and treatment may need to be begun gradually.

Several forms of topical retinoids exist, each with specific properties. An example is tretinoin.

Azelaic acid – This is an organic compound found in wheat, rye, and barley.

SOME NATURAL SOURCES OF SKIN LIGHTENING AGENTS

- Acerola cherry (Malpighia emarginata)
- Aloe vera[51]
- Apple cider vinegar
- Bitter root (Sophora flavescens)
- Black mulberry (Morus nigra)
- Breadfruit (Artocarpus incisus)
- Cantaloupe (Cucumis melo var. cantalupensis)

51   Ivana Binic, Viktor Lazarevic, Milanka Ljubenovic, Jelena Mojsa, and Dusan Sokolovic, "Skin Aging: Natural Weapons and Strategies," Evidence-Based Complementary and Alternative Medicine, vol. 2013, Article ID 827248, 10 pages, 2013. doi:10.1155/2013/827248

- Evening primrose (Oenothera biennis)[52]
- Kiwi fruit (Actinidia Chinensis)
- Kowhai (Sophora)
- Lemons or oranges (Citrus spp.) – ascorbic acid
- Licorice (Glycyrrhiza glabra)
- Milk and milk products—lactic acid
- Peony (Paeonia)
- Persimmon (Diospyros kaki) leaf
- Pineapple (Ananas comosus)
- Sea Grape (Coccoloba uvifera)
- Sugar beets (Beta vulgaris)
- Sugarcane (Saccharum officinarum)
- Turmeric (Curcuma longa)[53]
- Unripe grapes (Vitis vinifera)
- West Indian cherry (Acerola)

HOME-MADE SKIN LIGHTENING TREATMENTS

Find out how to make your own skin lightening creams at home, by visiting our recipes section ("Home-made Skin Care: skin lightening treatments" on page 291).

---

52   ibid.
53   ibid.

⟨⟩SKIN THERAPY: SKIN MICRONEEDLING

Surgical skin needling, sometimes called 'microneedling' or 'collagen induction therapy (CIT)', is very useful in the treatment of atrophic (depressed) facial acne scarring. It may have fewer side effects than laser treatments, particularly on darker skin types. Darker skin may be at risk of skin pigment changes with laser treatment, which is why skin needling is more appropriate for this type.

Skin needling can have dramatic results, improving the skin's appearance and giving it a natural, youthful glow. It can be used on the face, neck, abdomen and chest. The most common area for skin needling is the face, however; and it is unusual to have this treatment on the body. Any area of the face, except the nose, can be treated.

Skin needling/microneedling is a safe and effective technique for:

- accidental and traumatic scars
- follicular scarring ('enlarged pores')
- large scars such as C-Section scars
- skin rejuvenation
- stretch marks
- surgical scars on the face and body
- treating acne scars
- uneven skin texture
- wrinkles

The technique involves rolling the skin needling device over the treatment area. This punctures the skin multiple times with small needles. In some devices the needles jut from a cylindrical roller; in others they are attached to a 'wand' or 'pen'. The needles cause thousands of microscopic injuries to the skin. This is the most time-consuming part of the procedure, and may take up to two hours for treatment of the whole face.

Skin microneedling induces the body's own natural healing response, encouraging the damaged skin to begin a process of wound healing that is followed by regeneration and the production of new collagen. Collagen production continues for up to 12 months after the procedure. Depressed acne scars are improved, as well as general skin quality.

Before the procedure, the patient is injected with local anesthetic to numb the treatment areas. Clinicians may additionally give the patient inhaled anesthetic gas or some light intravenous anesthetic or sedation. The needling device is then repeatedly rolled over the treatment area.

Generally when the skin roller is used, one to three sessions are required for best results. With wands or pens, four to ten sessions are recommended. Note: it is claimed that skin needling which is performed with 3mm long needles produces significantly better results than needling performed with shorter needles.

Immediately following the treatment, the patient's skin may 'weep' or 'ooze' a little. The clinician will apply a dressing to absorb any liquid. This can generally be removed after 24 hours.

During the healing period, the clinician may recommend that the patient use topical retinoids (vitamin A creams) or other medical grade skin care products to boost the collagen-producing effects of skin needling.

Usually the patient will experience some redness and swelling of the skin for up to one week after the procedure, which may necessitate taking some time off work.

Treated skin may become infected if the patient experiences a cold-sore breakout during the healing period. Bacterial infection is also possible but improbable, particularly if the treated skin area is kept clean and the patient follows post-treatment instructions.

As no skin is actually removed, scarring is very rare. Milia (small white dots) may appear on the healing skin of some people; however these are easy to remove. Temporary acne-breakouts may also occur after skin needling.

Some brand names of skin needling include DermaPen® and Dermaroller® and EDermastamp®

Home skin needling kits are available. Their action is less aggressive (and effective) than clinical devices. Brand names include Dermawand™, Lotus™ and Skin-Inject™.

See also "Radiofrequency Microneedling" on page 231.

SKIN THERAPY: SKIN RESURFACING

Skin resurfacing includes such techniques as:
- exfoliation
- laser skin resurfacing
- mechanical peels such as microdermabrasion
- chemical peels

Exfoliation is a term that refers to the mechanical removal of dead skin cells on the epidermis, the skin's outermost surface. When these cells are sloughed away, younger, fresher skin cells are revealed and the skin appears smoother. This process should not be repeated more than every few days, as it also strips away the skin's natural barrier. After exfoliating, you should apply a good moisturizer.

Exfoliation can be done with an *exfoliating brush*. These small, plastic brushes, consisting of a head of natural bristles and a handle, are available at department stores and cosmetic stores. They can be used in the shower, or to 'dry brush' the skin. Use a circular motion when brushing. The body can be treated, from neck to toe. Be careful when using an exfoliating brush on the delicate skin of the face.

A *loofah or exfoliating glove* can also be used to exfoliate the body, but these are not recommended for the face, as they may be too rough.

Exfoliating scrubs are skin-friendly formulations that contain gently abrasive substances such as finely crushed fruit pits or coffee grounds, sugar, salt, baking soda or oatmeal. When rubbed onto the skin they act like sandpaper, loosening dead skin cells so that they can be rinsed away. Excellent natural exfoliating scrubs can be easily and cheaply made in your own home. See "Home-made Skin Care: exfoliating scrubs" on page 282.

Note: avoid buying scrubs that contain environmentally-destructive plastic micro-beads. Plastic also lacks other characteristics that are beneficial to the skin.

Laser skin resurfacing uses laser energy to remove skin cells from the outermost layer of skin. It can go further than removing only dead skin cells and actually vaporize living cells from the skin's surface. Laser energy can be precisely directed to remove skin layer by layer. Afterwards, as the skin heals, new cells and new collagen fibers are formed. The skin takes on a tighter, younger-looking appearance. This technique is ideal for treating skin discoloration, scars and wrinkles.

Dermabrasion and microdermabrasion are similar to laser skin resurfacing, except that instead of being vaporized by laser energy the outer layers of skin are mechanically abraded away. This is usually achieved by means of a high-speed rotary wheel with abrasive attachments such as a wire brush, diamond fraise, or sterilized sandpaper.

Chemical peels - The face can be treated by using an '*exfoliating mask*' formulation containing mild acids such as alpha-hydroxy acid and beta-hydroxy acid. Masks are creams that are applied to the face and allowed to remain for a while to act on the skin, before being washed off. See also "Home-made Skin Care: skin peels" on page 185.

Skin resurfacing can be used to treat the following conditions:

- Benign skin lesions.
- Blemishes and unevenly-textured skin.
- Pigmentation including freckles and hyperpigmentation.
- Sagging eyelids and aging facial features.
- Scars from acne, chicken pox, trauma or surgery.
- Sun-damaged skin.
- Wrinkles – especially fine wrinkles – around the eyes, lips, cheeks and forehead.

How it works

Inside the dermis (the deeper layer of the skin) are two sub-layers, both of which are constructed from long collagen and elastin fibers. These fibers become lax and overstretched as we age, and as sun damage accumulates. If the deepest layer becomes damaged, it results in scarring. The upper layer of the dermis, on the other hand, heals from wounds without scarring.

Skin resurfacing takes advantage of this fact. It removes the topmost skin layers down to the dermis. This triggers the growth of new skin cells and of those long, underlying collagen and elastin fibers. The outcome is smoother, firmer and healthier-looking skin.

SKIN THERAPY: SKIN TIGHTENING CREAMS

Commercially available creams may temporarily firm and tighten the skin of the face. The ingredients can include water, magnesium aluminium silicate (a naturally occurring mineral used as a thickener, which has very large molecules and cannot be absorbed by the skin), iron oxides (used to add color), sodium silicate (a buffering agent and pH adjuster, also a potential skin irritant), propylene glycol (a synthetic liquid substance that absorbs water), methylparaben and propylparaben (both of which are preservatives).

Molecules of collagen and elastin are too large to penetrate the skin's surface, so most of these 'skin firming' products exert their effect by forming a film on the skin's surface. This chemical film makes the skin look and feel tighter, and may smooth out the appearance of wrinkles for — it is claimed — up to ten hours.

These products are used by people who are seeking a quick and easy way to improve their appearance for a special occasion.

See also our recipes for home-made temporary skin tightening masks, page 296.

SKIN THERAPY: SKIN TIGHTENING INJECTIONS

Skin tightening injections are used to treat the face, neck and upper chest (décolletage). During the procedure, a substance called Poly-L Lactic Acid is injected into the deep layer of the skin.

The purpose of skin tightening injections is to counteract the aging process. As we age, our skin gradually loses its ability to manufacture collagen, and thus loses elasticity and volume. Poly-L lactic acid stimulates collagen production, thus restoring volume and tightness to the face. Skin tightening injections cannot be combined with other cosmetic procedures such as dermal filling. Generally the treatment involves two to three sessions, each about eight weeks apart.

Skin tightening injections can be used for:

- Adding lift, elasticity and volume to sunken cheeks.
- Improving the appearance of nose-to-mouth (nasolabial) grooves and creases at the corners of the mouth (marionettes).
- Plumping and firming wrinkles on the upper arms and thighs and on the backs of the hands.
- Reconstructing facial contours.
- Smoothing and firming large areas of wrinkles on the décolletage.

The procedure
Treatments generally take between 30 minutes to an hour, depending on the size of the area to be covered and the number of injections. The patient often has light, local anesthesia. The physician injects Poly-L lactic acid into the deep skin layers using a very thin needle, then massages it in. Needle puncture marks will be visible afterwards, but will have disappeared within 24 hours. It is not unusual to have temporary redness and minor bruising at the injection sites. This can be easily concealed with makeup. The treated area will be slightly swollen, but this swelling generally resolves overnight. Allergic reactions have been reported, but they are very rare.

The results

Results are not instantaneous and may take weeks or even months to develop, because the treatment relies on the skin's own natural repair processes, which work slowly. The improved volume and tightness can last up to one and a half years. Some patients have reported it lasting as long as two years. Eventually the body breaks down the Poly-L-Lactic and permanently replaces some of it with the body's own collagen.

Brand names of Poly-L-Lactic acid skin tightening injections include: Sculptra®, Sculptra Aesthetic®.

SKIN THERAPY: ULTRASOUND SKIN THERAPY

Ultrasound skin therapy is a non-surgical procedure. There are many applications for ultrasound in cosmetic medicine. They include:

- Exfoliating the skin, smoothing the texture and improving the evenness of skin color.
- Facial and body skin rejuvenating treatments.
- Reduction of stretch marks.
- Speeding up the healing and fading the discoloration of bruised areas.
- The pre- and post-operative treatment of cosmetic surgery patients to accelerate healing and recovery after procedures such as face lifts, tummy tucks, and liposuction.
- Treatment of contracture and scar tissue such as around breast implants.
- Ultrasound applied over certain creams contributes to greater effectiveness through deeper and more thorough penetration of the products.

The actions of ultrasound fall into four categories:

- The thermal effect; i.e. the benefits derived from heat directed the deeper tissues, which stimulates collagen production.
- The mechanical effect; i.e. the high-speed vibrations that act on the tissue like a micro-massage.
- The cavitation effect; i.e. the production of countless tiny droplets of oxygen, due to the vibrations.
- The biological effects, which include blood-vessel dilatation, improved blood flow and circulation, sonophoresis (an increased ability of the skin to absorb topical compounds), improved lymph flow, muscle relaxation, reduced inflammation, and pain relief.

Ultrasonic techniques have become common in daily life. Ultrasound has been used to shatter kidney stones, examine the fetus during pregnancy, study dolphins' language, train dogs, and clean contact lenses. Ultrasonic sound waves are the foundation of this technology and their frequency is higher than the level detected by the human ear.

Ultrasound skin treatment sessions may take about 30 to 45 minutes.

Dermapheresis or Sonophoresis

Stretch marks, fine lines, and sun-damaged skin are improved through dermapheresis or sonophoresis. These terms refer to the use of ultrasound in stimulating the deeper penetration of skincare formulations into the skin.

Researchers have found that ultrasound energy can temporarily change the structure of the outer skin layer, making it easier for topical applications to reach inner tissue layers. Rapid oscillations caused by ultrasound energy alter the permeability of the cell membranes and increases fibroblast activity and collagen formation.

Skin treatments become more effective when combined with ultrasound, because deep cleansing, exfoliation, and moisturizing are improved.

- Ultrasonic vibrations penetrate deep into pores and hair follicles to break up dead skin cells and oily blockages.
- The skin metabolism is boosted which causes lymph flow to increase so that waste products are removed more rapidly and effectively.
- The more waste products that are flushed away, the better the penetration and absorption of skincare products.
- Deep-tissue micro-massage improves skin tone, softness, and texture.

All combined, these factors create younger looking skin.

Treatment of scar tissue

Scar tissue and contracture are improved tremendously with ultrasound. It is thought that this is mainly due to the thermal effects of ultrasound working to loosen, stretch and re-orient collagen fibers. Treatment involves application of the ultrasound over the scarred areas followed by stretching and massaging exercises and the application of certain cream. Six to twelve sessions provide the best results, with improvements usually showing up after four sessions.

Combination ultrasound skin treatments

Some estheticians bring together the positive effects of microderm-abrasion, ultrasound technology, and potent creams.

Microdermabrasion removes the thickened and sun-damaged outer layer of skin.

Next, ultrasound application can deliver special creams deeper into the lower layers of the skin. In this way the ultimate effects of the creams are much more potent.

Multiple treatments are usually required, and this combination treatment is safe for all skin colors and types. The number and frequency of treatments depends on the patient's skin type and response to therapy. Improvements are usually seen by the fourth treatment.

Note that ultrasound skin therapy does not correct sun damage; and it doesn't reduce hollows caused by age-related fat loss. For these reasons it may be used in combination with other treatments, such as dermal fillers and laser resurfacing or a chemical peel. The full results may take a few months to appear.

Brand names of ultrasound devices include Ultherapy by Ulthera®.

SKIN THERAPY: ULTRAVIOLET RADIATION THERAPY

Ultraviolet radiation therapy is also known as phototherapy. It is well known that controlled exposure to ultraviolet radiation can aid in reducing the symptoms of chronic eczema or psoriasis. UV radiation therapy must be done strictly under medical supervision. Practitioners can rigorously monitor the treatment with the use of purposefully designed cabinets lined with fluorescent light tubes. The patient removes his or her clothes and stands in the cabinet to receive the ultraviolet radiation emitted by these tubes.

Depending on the severity of the skin disorder, up to 30 treatments may be required.

If you try ultraviolet radiation therapy on a do-it-yourself basis or without medical supervision, you run the risk of rapidly aging your skin and/or increasing your risk of skin cancer.

SKIN THERAPY: VACUUM SUCTION SKIN THERAPY

vacuum suction skin therapy is a non-surgical procedure. Cupping and vacuum massaging date back to ancient Egyptian times. In the 20th and 21st centuries, vacuum devices and simple mechanical devices that create suction have been used worldwide for treating acne, double chins, wrinkles and saggy skin.

Vacuum suction skin therapy boosts circulation and stimulates fibroblasts (cells that produce collagen), which firm the skin. It is also claimed to halt hair loss and stimulate hair growth.

This procedure is typically used to help decrease the appearance of cellulite, or to aid in microdermabrasion.

Vacuum Suction Cellulite Treatment

Cellulite, which is pocketed fat, may be effectively broken down with vacuum pressure. Vacuum suction skin therapy has been a standard treatment for cellulite reduction and firming up the muscles, because it increases blood supply, helps removes toxin and may boost immunity.

Cellulite forms as connective tissues that push fat cells upwards. This creates the dimpled look.

The vacuum suction procedure can have side effects. Importantly, the pressure for the vacuum should be controlled and monitored according to skin type, texture and condition. If used with too much pressure for too long, it can cause bruising, tenderness and even hematoma (swelling) and hemorrhage. Experts caution that frequent use of vacuum suction can actually *cause* skin laxity by damaging the underlying elastic fibers and collagen.

Handheld vacuum or suction massager brand names include Dirt Devil®, Celluless MD®.

Part 5:
Home-made
Skin Care Recipes

ABOUT MAKING YOUR OWN SKIN CARE FORMULATIONS

STORAGE AND LABELING

Always store your home-made skin care preparations in clean, sterilized containers that are lightproof. Label them clearly, e.g. 'Clay Skin Cleanser', and mark them with the date they were made.

SHELF LIFE

Additionally, if mixing your own skin care products make a little at a time and store under refrigeration. As a general rule, use them while they are still fresh; within two weeks.

EXTENDING SHELF LIFE

Your home-made product will need to be used while still fresh. Without preservatives it will have a short shelf life. If you'd rather use natural (or chemical) preservatives in your home-made skincare products, be aware of skin sensitivities.

Look for anti-fungal, anti-bacterial and anti-oxidant properties in your preservatives. Each ingredient in our 'Natural Preservatives' list possesses one or more properties. Make sure each property is included and mixes well with the others without including too much of any one property. Remember, large amounts of anti-microbials, anti-fungals etc. can be detrimental to your skin, so use as little as possible.

Always store products ingredients in a cool, dry, dim or dark place (preferably your refrigerator). A well-crafted moisturizer should last at least 4—6 weeks out of the refrigerator under normal conditions – that is, at less than 24° Celsius (75° Fahrenheit), stored in a dark, dry, clean place. It should last 3—6 months in and out of the refrigerator and touched only by clean fingers.

Always use sterile tools, containers and working spaces, and keep hands clean — both when making and using your products.

Store everything in clean, airtight containers, preferably made of a dark-colored plastic so that light cannot get in. You might wish to place all your 'wet' ingredients in one container – oils, butters, waxes, flower waters, aloe vera gel etc. – and your 'dry' ingredients, such as vitamin C powders, emulsifying wax beads, oatmeal, clay, sugar, powdered milk and herbal tea leaves in another.

NATURAL PRESERVATIVES

It is debatable how well natural preservatives actually work in cosmetics. Using them is no guarantee that your formula will not spoil when stored for long periods.

Some natural preservatives include:

* Cinnamon. This spice can inhibit the growth of yeast, mold, fungi and some bacteria. Some studies indicate that cinnamon works better as a preservative when it is combined with potassium sorbate. Add ¼ teaspoon of powdered cinnamon per 16 ounces (480 ml) of your formula. Do not use cinnamon oil, as it can be a skin irritant.

* Citric acid powder. Use 100% pure anhydrous citric acid. Add at 0.05%–0.3% to distilled water just after it has been boiled. Stir until the powder is dissolved and allow to cool before adding it to your formula. Do not use citric acid powder in sunscreen.

* Goldenseal root. This has been shown to inhibit the growth of fungi, mold, yeast and some bacteria. It is also traditionally used to combat eczema and other skin disorders. Soak ½ – 1 teaspoon per 12 oz (350 ml) distilled water mixture. Brew it as you would brew tea, and afterwards strain it through a fine strainer. You could alternatively brew it using a tea ball.

* Green tea. This is a potent antioxidant and can be bought in several forms. Use 0.5 – 3% green tea extract in your formula. If you buy the gel caps, cut or break the outer case and squeeze the liquid into your formula. If you prefer to buy green tea bags, allow one or two tea bags to soak in warm distilled water. Tea bags will not produce as powerful a preservative effect as the green tea extract. You can also use green tea leaf powder, at a concentration of 0.5 – 3%.

* Turmeric: The yellow pigment extracted from turmeric rhizomes exhibits strong antioxidant and antimicrobial activities. It does, however, add a yellow tint to your moisturizer, depending on how much you use.

* Rosemary. This fragrant herb is a is a natural antioxidant. Rosemary extract powder can be added to your formula at 0.1% to 0.5%. That is, about 0.3%, or ¼ teaspoon per 16 ounce (480 ml) of formula. Add rosemary oil extract at 0.1% to 0.5% to your oil mixture; i.e. approximately one drop per 1 ounce (30 ml) of your formula. Be wary of rosemary oil extract. Like other essential oils, it shouldn't be used on your skin without diluting it in a carrier oil.

* Vitamin E. This can be purchased in a form called 'T-50 mixed tocopherols'. It is a blend of natural tocopherols isolated from grain and seed oils such as soybean, sunflower, corn and canola. In this form it is a heat stable antioxidant that protects food and cosmetic products from oxidation. It only protects oil's shelf-life, and has no action against bacteria or mold. T-50 mixed tocopherols can be added to your formula at a rate of 0.04 − 0.5%.

* Other natural preservatives include neem oil, tea tree oil, honey, propolis, salt, vinegar and lemon juice.

* You can also extend your formula's shelf life by eliminating water as an ingredient and using only the oils, waxes and butters.

* Use your raw materials while they are fresh. Don't let your herbs get stale or your oils go rancid. Use your raw materials within three months and give each bottle of finished product no longer than a three-month shelf life.

A NOTE ON EMULSIFIERS:

Lotions and creams are created from a mixture of water and oils. Without the addition of emulsifiers, or alternatively the process of emulsification, the water and oils would separate. Think of emulsification as the glue that holds your ingredients together.

Emulsifying wax: For the first recipe below, you will need to use emulsifying wax. Emulsifying wax looks like white, waxy flakes which are easy to measure and melt. It makes the moisturizer cream less sticky and more stable than some of the alternative natural emulsifiers – that is, the water and oil in the cream are less likely to separate.

The ingredients for emulsifying wax are: Cetearyl Alcohol, Polysorbate 60, PEG-150 Stearate, and Steareth-20. These are synthetic substances manufactured in laboratories.

Home-made emulsifying wax: If you cannot get hold of emulsifying wax or if you'd rather not use synthetic substances, you can make your own home-made emulsifying wax. Mix together a combination of 80% beeswax, 10% borax, and 10% liquid lecithin.

Borax has fungicide, preservative, insecticide, herbicide, and disinfectant properties. Note, however, that it can also be a significant skin irritant!

You can also try swapping beeswax for vegetable waxes such as candelilla (Euphorbia antisyphilitica), carnauba (Copernicia prunifera), bayberry (Myrica spp.), or floral waxes.

Emulsifier-free moisturizers: If you wish to avoid both synthetic substances and borax, you can emulsify your moisturizer using a blender.

CARRIER OILS

Use a blended carrier oil base that includes vitamin E oil, tea tree oil, jojoba oil, avocado oil, olive oil, red raspberry seed oil, green tea, aloe vera or honey because of their naturally long lasting bacteria, mold and fungus fighting qualities.

Grape seed oil (Vitis vinifera)

Grape seed oil's smell is neutral and it makes a moisturizer with a pleasant texture which absorbs well without feeling greasy. It is an excellent emollient, and does not clog pores or give you pimples. It has a good shelf life, it is widely available from any grocery store and it is (relatively) cheap.

Jojoba oil (Simmondsia chinensis)

This shares many of grape seed oil's qualities including emollient properties, and it is a valuable source of wax esters. It is, however, more expensive than grape seed oil.

Castor oil (Ricinus communis)

This oil is also odor free and has a good shelf life, plus it has the advantage of containing lots of ricinoleic acid. Castor oil has a useful anti-inflammatory effect, but it gives your home-made cream an unpleasantly heavy, sticky feel if there's too much of it.

If you are suffering from an eczema outbreak you can combine castor oil with grape seed oil. Measure 1/3 cup grape seed oil and add enough castor oil to make ½ cup. This mixture may help reduce inflammation.

Coconut oil (Cocos nucifera)

This is safe, gentle and effective. It is also anti-oxidant, emollient, antibacterial and antimicrobial, though it is considered to be somewhat comedogenic. If you have a tendency to get clogged pores and blackheads, coconut oil might exacerbate the problem.

Argan oil (Argania spinosa)

This carrier oil is used to hydrate and soften skin. With its high vitamin E and fatty acid content, argan oil is an emollient that absorbs easily and is non-greasy and non-irritating, which makes it a great natural moisturizer.

Safflower seed oil (Carthamus tinctorius)

This is a natural, non-fragrant emollient carrier oil.

Wheat germ Oil (Triticum aestivum)

Wheat germ oil penetrates the skin to soothe eczema and irritations. It also aids in wound healing and can improve the appearance of scar tissue. It is dark yellow to orange in color, with a fairly strong odor. This oil is rich in vitamin E, as well as vitamins B1, B2, B3, B6, and A. It contains a number of beneficial minerals to nourish the skin.

Rice Bran Oil (Oryza sativa)

Rice bran oil is loaded with vitamin E. It can provide relief from eczema, psoriasis or dermatitis and is non-greasy.

Avocado Oil (Persea americana)

Always use unrefined avocado oil. It contains high concentrations of vitamins A, D and E, is effective for eczema relief and is beneficial for dry, dehydrated or aging skin. Because this oil is somewhat heavy, it is suggested you mix it with a lighter oil such as sweet almond.

Sweet Almond Oil (Prunus dulcis)

Sweet almond oil is light and finely textured. It is easily absorbed and helps to leave the skin soft and smooth. An emollient and a moisturizer, sweet almond oil is rich in Vitamins A and E and helps relieve skin irritation.

COLD- PRESSED OILS LAST LONGER

Dried herbs and cold-pressed, refrigerated oils may last longer. Mechanically extracted oils will stay active and fresh no longer than six months, even when refrigerated. It's not just about whether the lotion spoils or keeps. We need the fatty acids and vitamins in the lotion to nourish our skin. If a lotion loses its freshness, it will be useless or even cause free radical damage and age our skin prematurely.

WATER

Always use distilled water or boiled-and-cooled water. Products made without water last longer. The least amount of water you use, the better.

BEWARE OF ESSENTIAL OILS

Avoid adding essential oils to your skin care preparations, as many of them can cause sun sensitivity (phototoxicity), otherwise also known as photosensitization. The agent in the oil causing this sun sensitivity is 'bergaptene'. Skin that has become over-sensitive to sunlight is more easily damaged by sunburn.

The main oils causing phototoxicity are those from the citrus family, when they are extracted by direct expression and without distillation. There are, however, some oils — like lemon — which still remain phototoxic even after distillation.

Oils like bergamot, lime and bitter orange are severely phototoxic when used undiluted, but the sun sensitizing effect is decreased when they are used in very low dilutions.

Other pure, natural essential oils can also contain potential skin irritants such as terpene, methanol and limonene[54].

---

54   *J Toxicol Environ Health B Crit Rev. 2013;16(1):17-38. doi: 10.1080/10937404.2013.769418. Safety evaluation and risk assessment of d-Limonene. Kim YW, Kim MJ, Chung BY, Bang du Y, Lim SK, Choi SM, Lim DS, Cho MC, Yoon K, Kim HS, Kim KB, Kim YS, Kwack SJ, Lee BM.*

AVOID FRAGRANCES

Many commercial skin-care products contain added fragrance. Most fragrant ingredients give off their scent by way of a volatile reaction, which almost always causes irritation of the skin and some inflammation. Research has shown that fragrances in skin-care products are among the most common causes of sensitizing and allergic reactions.

Even if your skin doesn't look irritated or inflamed, the fragrance might still be a problem. The outermost layer of skin (the epidermis) generally hides the fact that it's being irritated by showing no obvious reaction.

Below the surface, irritating ingredients can cause collagen to break down, obstruct the skin's capacity to fight environmental damage, and impede the skin's capacity to heal. All this can be happening in the lower layers of skin without any visible signs on the surface!

The irritant reaction you don't see or feel is nonetheless harming your skin's capacity to decrease wrinkles, retain elasticity and appear youthful. For people with sensitive skin, and especially those with rosacea or acne, fragrances irritate the skin so severely that the reaction *will* show up on the surface. Fragrance of any kind (including natural essential oils) should be strictly avoided.

ROSE FLOWER WATER

There is are a couple of exceptions to the above rule. One is rose flower water. If you really want to add fragrance to your home-made skin care preparations, choose pure rose flower water.

Since the dawn of history, rose flower water has been used in both skin care and cookery. Rose flower water is a gentle emollient with anti-inflammatory properties. Most other natural flower waters may contain irritants – orange blossom water ('neroli') and lavender flower water, for example, contain terpenes and methanol.

Flower waters, also known as hydrosols, hydroflorates, or distillates, are produced by steam-distilling plant materials. They are like essential oils but not nearly as concentrated.

Note that many commercial 'floral waters' are manufactured either from synthetic compounds or by mixing water with essential oils.

They have a pleasant fragrance, but lack the beneficial constituents of true rose flower water, and may cause skin reactions.

Rose flower water is a water extraction of rose oil and tannins from rose petals. The traditional (and best) variety of rose for this purpose is *Rosa gallica officinalis*, whose common names include the Gallic Rose, the French Rose, the Rose of Provins, the Red Damask Rose and the Apothecary's Rose. This rose is one of the most celebrated of all ancient roses.

HOME-MADE SKIN CARE: ROSE FLOWER WATER

Making your own rose flower water

Since you are going to be applying the rose water to your skin, it is important to make sure the petals you use have not been sprayed with chemicals. The pesticides and fungicides used on roses will not necessarily be removed by washing, and they will end up on your skin, which can be harmful.

Either buy dried organic rose petals or pick your own unsprayed roses from your garden. If you are not growing the Apothecary's Rose, any sweet-scented rose will do; it just won't have the rich and heady fragrance that made *Rosa gallica officinalis* so famous throughout the ages. The color of the rose petals will tint the water pale pink or pale gold, or even amber.

The best time to pick the flowers is very early in the morning, when they are fully hydrated, before the sun's rays start to dry them out. Pull off the petals, place them gently in a colander or sieve and rinse them under clean tap water.

The traditional method of making rose water is by distillation. Water extracts can also be made by infusion. Herbal tea is an example of a water extract made this way.

Home-made rose flower water - distilled

Equipment:
- An oven-safe glass or ceramic bowl
- A heatproof pot or casserole dish with a glass or metal lid. This pot should be big enough for the bowl to fit inside
- A brick or metal rack that fits in the bottom of the pot or casserole dish
- Fresh or dried organic rose petals, rinsed clean
- Distilled water
- Baggies filled with ice cubes and sealed.

Instructions:
- Place the pot or casserole dish on top of your stove, with the brick or rack inside.
- Add rose petals, up to the height of the brick or rack.
- Pour in enough distilled water to just cover the rose petals.
- Place the empty bowl on the rack, turn on the stove and heat the water to a slow simmer.
- Place the lid upside down on the pot. Place a baggie or two filled with ice cubes into the inverted lid.
- The steam from the simmering water, laden with essence of roses, will rise and meet the cold lid. It will condense and run down the lid until it drips into the bowl.
- When the ice in the baggies melts, simply remove the watery baggies from the lid and replace them with fresh icy ones. This saves you from having to lift off the lid to pour the water away. Lifting the lid means you would lose some of your rosewater-filled steam.
- When all the water has simmered away out of the pot, what remains in the bowl will be pure rose flower water.

Home-made rose flower water - infused

Distillation is the best and most traditional way to make rose flower water, but you can also make it by infusion. This method is a little easier.

Equipment:
- A heatproof pot or casserole dish with a glass or metal lid.
- 2 cups fresh or dried organic rose petals, rinsed clean.
- Distilled water - enough to cover the rose petals when they are in the dish.
- A sterilized strainer.
- A sterilized glass jar with a lid.
- Labels and pens.

Instructions:
- Preheat your oven to 300° Fahrenheit (150° Celsius).
- Place the rose petals into the casserole dish.
- Bring the distilled water to a boil and pour it over the rose petals.
- Cover the dish with the lid, place it into the oven and cook for 20 minutes.
- After that time has elapsed, turn the oven off but leave the dish inside.
- When the dish has cooled to the point at which you can touch it, take it out.
- Strain the water into the sterile glass jar.
- Label it with the name of the contents and the date.

Shelf life of rose flower water

Unpreserved rose water will keep for about a week at room temperature or for up to a month in the refrigerator. To keep it longer, freeze it.

How to use rose flower water

- Pour rose flower water into a spray bottle and use it as a cooling mist or body perfume.
- Use it as an ingredient in your home-made skin moisturizers and cleansers
- Make rose water skin lotion: When rose water is blended with glycerin it makes a silky, skin-smoothing lotion. Mix together three parts rosewater with one part vegetable glycerin.

HOME-MADE SKIN CARE: HIBISCUS FLOWER WATER

Another flower water that may be used in home-made skin care preparations is hibiscus. Unlike rose flower water, this is not a fragrant additive.

Some pure flower water extracts such as Hibiscus sabdariffa flower extract are said to possess anti-oxidant and emollient properties, and to inhibit elastin degradation to maintain skin elasticity. Hibiscus flower water is used to firm and tone the skin, smooth the appearance of fine lines and unclog pores.

Home-made hibiscus flower water

Ingredients:
- 1 cup dried hibiscus flowers
- 8 cups water

Instructions:
- Combine ingredients in a large saucepan.
- Bring to a boil, then turn off the heat.
- Allow mixture to steep for 30 minutes.
- Strain into a sterile, lidded jar, label and refrigerate.

Use and store hibiscus flower water according to the instructions for rose flower water.

HOME-MADE SKIN CARE: SOAP-FREE SKIN CLEANSERS

CHICKPEA FLOUR SKIN CLEANSER

Chickpeas are also known as gram, garbanzo bean, Egyptian pea, ceci, cece or chana. Chick pea flour, also known as 'besan', is an excellent cleanser for very oily skin. You can buy it in most Asian groceries or health food stores. Mix it to your desired consistency with distilled or boiled-and-cooled water, aloe vera gel, rose flower water, hibiscus flower extract or another appropriate ingredient of your choice and apply in the same way as clay skin cleanser (see below) or orris root powder cleanser.

CLAY SKIN CLEANSER

Clay draws oil and dirt from the skin and may soothe inflammation. You can use it as a face mask or as a daily face wash.

There are various types of skin cleansing clays including red, green or white clay, ghassoul (also called rhassoul), Fullers' Earth or healing earth. You can mix clay with distilled or boiled-and-cooled water or other ingredients such as aloe vera gel, rose flower water, hibiscus flower extract. Do not add many different ingredients simultaneously. Try only one thing at a time to gauge how your skin reacts to it.

If your skin has a tendency to be dry, add a few drops of oil. To enhance antibacterial properties, add a drop of tea tree oil, a teaspoon of manuka honey or a splash of apple cider vinegar.

To use, apply the mixture to your face, leave it on for a few minutes, then rinse. Do not allow it to dry out on your skin. Do not use clay if you are allergic to nickel, because clay may contain traces of it.

You can use clay as a mask for body and hair as well, particularly ghassoul. See page 297 for more information about Fullers' Earth.

Clay as a cleanser works especially well on oily or combination skins. Nonetheless, there is a clay for every skin type —

- *For oily skin:* ghassoul / rhassoul (Moroccan lava clay), green clay, bentonite clay, kaolin clay or Fuller's Earth.
- *For sensitive skin:* white clay, red clay.
- *For dry skin:* red clay.
- *For dull, tired, or devitalized skin:* pink clay.

REFRESHING SKIN CLEANSER

This mixture cleans and refreshes your skin. It does not dry out the skin and it leaves no residue. The baking soda has a gentle exfoliant action and the aloe soothes and heals. Note, however, it is not pH balanced; the baking soda makes it a little alkaline.

Ingredients:
- ½ cup water
- 2 tablespoon aloe vera gel
- 2 tablespoons vegetable glycerin
- 2 tablespoons baking soda
- ½ teaspoon xanthan gum (to thicken)

Optional additives:
- 2 tablespoons witch hazel
- 2 tablespoons raw honey
- 1 tsp calendula extract
- 1 teaspoon chamomile extract
- 1 teaspoon green tea extract
- 1 teaspoon ginger extract
- 15 drops coconut oil
- 15 drops almond oil

Instructions:
- Mix together your chosen ingredients.
- To thicken use ½ tsp xanthan gum whizzed in with a blender.
- When all is well-blended, pour the mixture into a clean bottle and seal with an airtight lid.
- Label the bottle.
- Store in refrigerator to prolong shelf life.
- To use, simply rub it over your skin, then rinse off with warm water and pat dry with a soft towel.

SOOTHING SKIN CLEANSER

Fragrant rosewater adds a luxurious touch to this gentle cleanser. Never use essential oils on your skin – despite being all-natural, they can cause phototoxicity and irritation. All perfumes can be irritants , even natural rose, so if you find it's a problem for you, substitute distilled water or boiled and cooled water. Natural rosewater is, nonetheless, very beneficial to the skin.

Ingredients:
- ¼ cup aloe vera gel
- 2 tablespoons almond oil
- 2 tablespoons natural rosewater
- 1 tablespoon soapwort extract[55]
- 5-10 drops coconut oil
- 3-5 drops or 1 capsule vitamin E oil (optional)

Instructions:
- Mix all ingredients together and store in container with tight fitting lid.
- To use: wet the face, apply in small circles and rub in for 30 seconds, then wash off with warm water.
- The water and oil may separate, so shake the container well before use.

RAW ORGANIC HONEY SKIN CLEANSER
Raw organic honey, especially Manuka honey, is an extremely mild cleanser with antibacterial and moisturizing benefits. Simply apply, leave on for a few minutes and rinse.

ORRIS ROOT POWDER SKIN CLEANSER

---

55   Soapwort extract is available from online stores and cosmetics stores. Note: soapwort (Saponaria officinalis) is a useful and pretty plant, easily grown in the garden.

The orris plant is botanically known as *Iris germanica, Iris florentina*, or *Iris pallida*. Orris root powder is moisturizing, very gentle on the skin and pleasantly scented like violets.

Mix the powder with distilled or boiled-and-cooled water (or aloe vera gel, rose flower water, hibiscus flower extract) and use it to cleanse your skin in the same way as the clay mixtures.

Browse online herb shops to find orris root powder, or ask in drugstores or pharmacies. You could also grow your own in the garden!

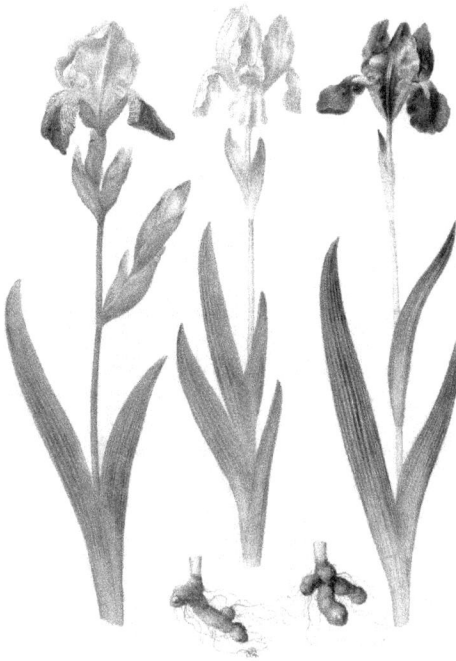

Iris germanica

HOME-MADE SKIN CARE: SKIN MOISTURIZERS

Dry skin is caused by a loss of water in the upper layer of the skin. The most effective way to moisturize your skin is to use a product that contains occlusive, humectant, and/or emollient ingredients. Apply your moisturizer in the morning, over the top of your vitamin C serum. Sunscreen may be applied over the top of your moisturizer.

Preservatives in moisturizers help prevent bacterial growth. Other ingredients in commercial moisturizers may include vitamins, minerals, plant extracts and fragrances.

MOISTURIZERS FOR DIFFERENT SKIN TYPES

- For *normal skin* light, non-greasy water-based moisturizers often contain lightweight oils, such as cetyl alcohol, or silicone-derived ingredients, such as cyclomethicone.

- For treating *skin dryness*, typical moisturizers are heavier, oil-based formulae that contain ingredients such as antioxidants or grape seed oil.

- For *very dry, cracked skin*, petrolatum-based products are usually used, as they are more lasting than creams and are more effective in preventing water evaporation.

- For *oily skin*, moisturizers can still be useful after activities causing skin dryness, such as washing, or application of other skin care products. Water-based moisturizers that are specifically non-comedogenic are preferable for oily skin, as there is less risk of blackhead or whitehead formation.

- Appropriate moisturizers to keep *aging skin* soft and well hydrated are oil-based ones that contain petrolatum as the base, along with antioxidants or alpha hydroxy acids to combat wrinkles.

- On *sensitive skin* (which is susceptible to irritation, redness, itching or rashes), it is preferable to use moisturizers which contain soothing ingredients such as chamomile or aloe. Avoid potential allergens/irritants such as fragrances, dyes or acids.

MAKING YOUR OWN SKIN MOISTURIZERS

Some examples of natural skin care ingredients for home-made moisturizers include jojoba oil, vegetable glycerin, rose hip oil, shea butter, beeswax, aloe vera, tea tree oil and chamomile. These ingredients can be combined to cater specifically to your skin type or skin condition.

BASIC MOISTURIZER (WITH EMULSIFYING WAX)

Equipment:
- Hand-held stick blender: These are easier to use and clean than standard bench-top blenders. More importantly, they permit you to blend smaller quantities. If you do not have a stick blender you can use a small whisk, but it takes a lot more time and energy.
- Cookery thermometer (optional).
- Container: Preferably, the container for your moisturizer ought to be a 450g (16 oz) wide-mouthed glass jar. If you do not have access to such a container, you can use a soft, plastic squeeze bottle such as a honey squeeze bottle or tomato sauce squeeze bottle. Your finished skin cream will be thick, and you will need an opening wide enough to let you scoop it out.

Ingredients:
For the most basic moisturizer you only need four ingredients:
- ½ cup grape seed oil (or carrier oil of your choice: see above)
- ¼ cup emulsifying wax (available from soap-making suppliers; this binds the oil and water into a smooth cream).
- ¾ cup distilled or boiled-and-cooled water
- ¼ tsp pure liquid vitamin E (this powerful antioxidant acts as a preservative as well as helping protect your skin against UV damage and assisting in in the healing of damaged tissue).

To this basic formula, you can add optional extras such as:

- 1 tbsp vegetable glycerin (add this to the water and be precise in your measurements; too much makes your moisturizer sticky).

- 12-15 drops of rose flower water

Instructions:
- Thoroughly wash and sterilize all your measuring cups, bowls, containers and tools. Cleanliness leads to longer shelf life. To sterilize recycled PET containers, wash them with hot water and soap then swish a little rubbing alcohol around inside them, drip out the excess and let it evaporate. Glass containers can easily be sterilized in a hot dishwasher or by immersing the jar in a saucepan of cold water and gradually bringing it to the boil. Simmer for 15 minutes.
- In a small container such as a stainless steel measuring cup, combine emulsifying wax and carrier oil.
- Heat over a saucepan of simmering water till the wax melts, stirring until ingredients are thoroughly combined.
- Over the same pot of simmering water, but in a separate container, warm the water so the oil and water reach approximately the same temperature.
- Slowly drip the oil mix into the hot water while blending rapidly with the stick blender until the oil and water are thoroughly emulsified.
- After it cools down to 48°C 120°F (about the temperature of a tepid cup of coffee) you can blend in the optional additives.
- Pour the mixture into your container(s) before it gets a chance to thicken.
- Storage: Vitamin E acts as a preservative, but even so, it will not stop your home-made moisturizer from going rancid and moldy if it is not used up while still fresh. Some people add a few drops of Germall® to their recipe; however others claim that this antimicrobial product contains skin irritants. The answer is to make small quantities and use them up very quickly. Or, instead of putting the cream in one big jar, use several small ones and store all the extras in the refrigerator.

Make sure you take a look at the moisturizer before you apply it. If it looks or smells 'off', throw it out.

BASIC MOISTURIZER (WITHOUT EMULSIFIERS)

This is a more natural formula than the recipe above, because it uses no synthetic emulsifiers. It is perhaps not quite as easy to make because you need to get the mixing technique just right. If you follow the instructions and use good quality ingredients you should be successful.

Other advantages include the fact that it is almost edible so fits with that old saying, 'you shouldn't put anything on your skin that you wouldn't put in your mouth.' The high oil content makes it great for dry skins or skin conditions. You only need to use a tiny amount so it lasts for ages and it has a pleasing look and feel.

Disadvantages are that it can be more expensive to make than many other creams which have a high amount of water and little infused oil or butters and it will not last indefinitely as it has no preservative. Also it can be too rich for some people who like very light creams or have oily skins.

One of the ingredients is an herbal infusion. To make a herbal infusion, place one heaped tablespoon of dried chopped herbs or petals into a mug. Fill the mug to the brim with 9 fluid ounces (250 ml) of boiling water. Allow this 'tea' to stand and brew for 10 minutes, then strain out the plant material, keep the liquid infusion, and allow it to cool before using it. Herbs that can be used include yarrow, thyme, rosemary, mint, mallow, calendula and chamomile.

Equipment:
- Blender: The emulsification process requires a good quality benchtop blender. You don't need the most expensive blender on the market, but it does need to be capable of running efficiently for a long time at a fairly low speed, without stopping due to overheating.

- Bain Marie or double boiler: You need to melt your waxes, butter and oils over a gentle, moist heat.
- Spatula: Required for scraping down the sides of the blender.
- Container: Preferably, the container for your moisturizer ought to be a 450g (16 oz) wide-mouthed glass jar. If you do not have access to such a container, you can use a soft, plastic squeeze bottle such as a honey squeeze bottle or tomato sauce squeeze bottle. Your finished skin cream will be thick, and you will need an opening wide enough to let you scoop it out.

Ingredients:
- 250ml (8oz) herbal infusion (or 200 ml (6oz) herbal infusion mixed with 50ml (2oz) pure aloe vera juice)
- 1 tsp vegetable glycerin
- 175ml (6oz) carrier oil
- 75g (3oz) coconut oil
- 25g (1oz) beeswax
- 5ml (85 drops) vitamin E oil

Instructions:
- Melt the beeswax and butters in a bain marie or double boiler at a low temperature, then add the liquid oils and mix until well blended.
- Pour the oil mixture into your blender and allow it to cool.
- While the oils/waxes/butters are cooling, mix together the 'waters'.
- After a few minutes, depending on the room temperature, the oils should turn from translucent and runny to opaque and thick.
- Don't let it over-solidify. It should still move a bit when you pick up the jug. If any has congealed on the sides, scrape it down with a spatula.
- The mixture should be opaque, but not solid all the way through.

- Turn the blender on to a fairly low speed and begin to pour in the waters in a slow trickle.
- This is the process of emulsification. (It's the same process used to make home-made mayonnaise.)
- If the mixture becomes stuck in the blender turn off the machine, scrap down the sides with a spatula and turn it back on again. Keep adding the waters bit by bit until it is all blended in, forming a smooth cream that is thick but still able to be poured.
- Stir in the vitamin E by hand and pour your moisturizer into the clean, prepared jars. Spoon in the final scrapings. You can use a chopstick to swirl the top decoratively, if you wish.
- This moisturizer contains no preservatives but should still last up to three months if stored in the refrigerator. To ensure a longer shelf-life, add a preservative, either natural or synthetic.

HOME-MADE SKIN CARE: SKIN SERUMS

VITAMIN C SERUM

Vitamin C is the only antioxidant that is proven to stimulate the synthesis of collagen, the protein that makes the skin elastic. Elasticity stops wrinkles from forming. Your body's natural collagen production decreases as you age. Sun exposure will also accelerate the decrease in collagen.

Studies have shown that vitamin C helps to minimize fine lines, scars, and wrinkles, effectively reversing age-related skin damage. Vitamin C also lightens age spots and sun spots. It is a powerful antioxidant and reduces the number of sun-damaged skin cells, it can reverse UV damage like pigmented spots and fine lines. This wonderful vitamin can also reduce inflammation. Regular use of a good vitamin C serum can make the skin 'glow'.

The extraction of vitamin C from plant materials requires an assortment of chemicals and equipment, as well as some training in chemistry. This is why some people create home-made face masks from fruits that are high in vitamin C, such as kiwi fruit, guavas, strawberries, papaya and citrus fruits.

Alternatively, you can use manufactured L-Ascorbic Acid powder as the active ingredient in your home-made serum.

L-Ascorbic Acid (also known as ascorbic acid or L-ascorbate) is the only form of vitamin C that you should look for in commercial skin care products. There are many skin care products on the market today that tout vitamin C derivatives as an ingredient (magnesium ascorbyl phosphate or ascorbyl palmitate, for example), but L-ascorbic acid is the only useful form of vitamin C in commercial skin care products.

After vitamin C has been moistened by being added to a serum or cream, it begins to lose its potency. It is unstable, and has a very short shelf life. The shelf life decreases more rapidly if it is exposed to light, so store your home-made vitamin C serum in a dark amber or dark blue glass bottle and keep it in a cool cupboard or your refrigerator. Make a small batch at a time and use it only for 3-5 days. This is a bit more time-consuming, but it is one way to ensure your serum is potent.

As an option, if you have access to a processing machine - such as a high-quality spice grinder - you can grind L-ascorbic acid powder to the fineness of dust. Store this dust in a small, sealed container.

When you want to use it as a serum, shake about a quarter of a teaspoon of vitamin C dust into the cupped palm of your hand, add a couple of drops of a carrier oil, and dabble the mixture with a fingertip until it is blended. Then apply all of it to your skin.

Once the vitamin C powder has been moistened, use it all up - because it cannot be stored without losing its potency.

Vitamin C serum can also be used on the backs of your hands. As we age, sun spots often appear in this area. Note that vitamin C may initially cause some irritation. It is normal to experience a slight tingling sensation when you apply it, but if the sensation is more like 'burning' immediately wash it off. To dilute the serum so that it is more suitable for sensitive skin, simply add more water and/or glycerin.

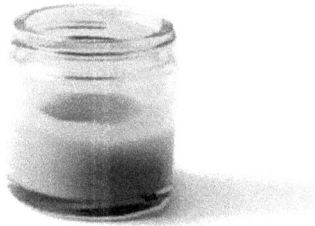

HOME-MADE VITAMIN C SERUM

Ingredients:

- 1 teaspoon natural L-ascorbic acid (vitamin C) powder
- 1 teaspoon distilled water
- small amber or dark glass bottle with tight-fitting stopper.

Optional ingredients:
- 1 teaspoon vegetable glycerin
- ⅛ teaspoon pure liquid vitamin E
- pure rose flower water or hibiscus flower extract

Instructions:

- Mix ingredients in a small bowl until the granules are dissolved.
- If you choose not to use glycerin, flower water/extract or vitamin E, add an extra teaspoon of water so that your serum is not too strong.
- Pour the serum into a dark glass bottle.

To use:

Apply vitamin C to the skin in the morning after cleansing. Let the serum soak in before applying your daily moisturizer, followed by a sunscreen if you'll be going outdoors or working near a bright window.

This recipe makes enough to last 3-5 days. To ensure that your stored home-made vitamin C serum remains optimized to benefit your skin, test it with a pH test strip (available from drugstores and pharmacies). Your serum's pH should be about 3.5.

RETINOL SERUM

Retinol is a derivative of vitamin A, and is a popular ingredient in many commercial skin care products. Retinol's stronger cousin is Retin-A (tretinoin). If your skin is too sensitive to use Retin-A, retinol is an excellent alternative.

Skin responds retinol because the molecules of vitamin A are tiny enough to pass into the lower layers of skin, lies our collagen and elastin. Retinol is proven to improve mottled pigmentation, fine lines and wrinkles, skin texture, skin tone and color, as well as your skin's hydration levels. Another cousin of retinol is retinyl palmitate. If your skin care product contains retinyl palmitate, you will need to use more of it than one that contains retinol to get the same effect.

We all know that eating carrots is a good way to boost our levels of vitamin A. It would be great if we could use carrots as a source of retinol (vitamin A) for the skin; however, retinol cannot be extracted directly from carrots. Carrots contain beta-carotene, which is a precursor of vitamin A, but it is not the same. The beta-carotene from carrots is converted into vitamin A by the human body. Therefore as the basis of our home-made retinol serum, we must use Vitamin A that has been obtained in a laboratory.

If you cannot obtain retinol or Retin-A, you can use retinyl palmitate. Retinyl palmitate is a combination of retinol (pure vitamin A) and palmitic acid. Research shows it to be effective as an antioxidant and skin-cell regulator.[56]

Retinyl palmitate is one of the primary antioxidants found naturally in skin.[57] It is approved by the FDA as a food additive, as an over-the-counter drug, and a prescription drug. To achieve premarket approval, the FDA requires extensive and rigorous testing. Retinyl palmitate has been shown in UVB exposure studies to offer sun protection all by itself, and it is a potent antioxidant.[58]

If you wish, you can use an exfoliating facial scrub before applying retinol, to remove excess dead skin cells and permit better absorption. Alternative methods for exfoliation include wearing a pair of special exfoliating gloves, which are relatively cheap and usually available from druggists/pharmacies. Do not, however, exfoliate more than twice a week, or you risk skin damage. Formulations for home-made facial scrubs can be found in "Home-made Skin Care Recipes" on page 250.

HOME-MADE RETINOL SERUM

Ingredients:

---

56   *European Journal of Medical Research, September 2001, pages 391–398; and Journal of Investigative Dermatology, September 1997, pages 301–305*

57   *Toxicology and Industrial Health, May 2006, pages 181-191.*

58   *International Journal of Pharmaceutics, October 2007, pages 181–189; and Journal of Investigative Dermatology, November 2003, pages 1,163–1,167*

- Retinol liquid or retinyl palmitate liquid drops (or vitamin A tablets or capsules. Available from drugstores/pharmacies, supermarkets or online).
- A gentle, hypoallergenic facial moisturizer (such as Cetaphil®, which contains no hydroquinone or parabens and will not interfere with vitamin A's action).
- Dry milk powder for added texture.

Instructions:
- Place two teaspoonsful of moisturizer in a small bowl. .
- Add one-quarter of a teaspoon of liquid retinol and mix well. If your retinol is in tablet form, use a mortar and a pestle to crush it to powder first. If it's in capsule form, cut the casing and shake out the powder. If it is in gel form, prick a hole in the capsule and squeeze out the gel.
- If you wish to add texture to the serum, mix in some powdered milk a little at a time until the serum reaches your desired consistency.

To use:
Apply generously to face. Massage well using your fingertips, until skin is well saturated. If using the milk-textured serum, apply to face and leave for thirty minutes to penetrate the skin. Rinse with warm water and pat dry.

Storage:
Make small batches at a time. Pour into clean, sterile containers, labeled and dated, and seal. Keep refrigerated and use within two weeks.

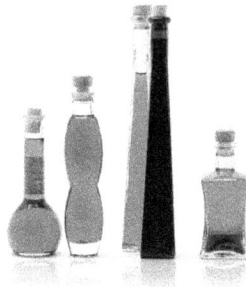

VITAMIN E AND VITAMIN B SERUMS

A 2010 study reported, 'Daily use of a facial lotion containing niacinamide (niacin and niacinamide are forms of Vitamin B3), panthenol (vitamin B5), and tocopheryl acetate (vitamin E) improved skin tone and texture...'[59]

59   Indian Journal of Dermatology, Venereology and Leprology 2010, Volume : 76, Issue : 1, Page : 20-26 The effects of a daily facial lotion containing vitamins B3 and E and provitamin B5 on the facial skin of Indian women: A randomized, double-blind trial. Hemangi R Jerajani, Haruko Mizoguchi, James Li, Debora J Whittenbarger, Michael J Marmor. Department of Dermatology, L.T.M. Medical College, L.T.M. General Hospital, Mumbai, India. 2 The Procter and Gamble Company, Sharon Woods Technical Center, Cincinnati, OH, USA DOI:

Vitamin E is a common ingredient in skin care products because of its antioxidant and healing characteristics.

The recommended usage rate in skincare formulations is 0.5 − 5% Buy a bottle of vitamin E capsules. You can snip open the capsules and squeeze out the contents to use directly on your skin. Wheatgerm oil is high in vitamin E and essential fatty acids; it can be mixed with the contents of vitamin E capsules and used as a moisturizer or carrier oil.

Niacinamide is the active form of Vitamin B3. Topical application of niacinamide has a number of benefits including:

- Improving the appearance of aging skin
- Improving the appearance of photodamaged skin
- Increasing skin moisturization.
- Improving skin texture
- Fading hyperpigmented spots
- Improving red blotchiness
- Reducing the severity of fine wrinkles
- Stimulating collagen synthesis
- Encouraging the production of ceramide, a lipid compound that contributes to the functional and structural integrity of the skin barrier. By improving barrier integrity, niacinamide may help the skin resist external irritants.
- Effectively reduce the skin's rate of sebum excretion, which in turn leads to an improvement of acne.

Niacinamide powder can be purchased from druggists/pharmacies and online. If you cannot obtain the powder, buy the tablets and crush them as finely as possible.

Niacinamide is soluble in water, so to make a basic skincare lotion mix it with pure rose flower water, or cooled green tea, or glycerin. Stir or shake until it is completely dissolved.

A few pinches or a teaspoonful can be added to any of your home-made skincare products, as long as you add it to the water-based ingredients first, and dissolve it thoroughly before you add any oils.

The pH of niacinamide is important when using it in skincare products. Do not use it in acidic formulations. When it is mixed with acids it hydrolyzes, forming nicotinic acid, a skin irritant. The final pH of your niacinamide-containing formula should be no lower than about pH 6.

Never use more than 4% niacinamide in your skincare formulations, because it can cause flushing (skin redness). Begin with a concentration of 1% and, after you have used this for a couple of weeks, increase the amount to 2%. Continue this gradual increase until in about six weeks you should be able to tolerate 4%.

Research carried out by cosmetics company Procter & Gamble and reported in 2012 discovered that skin moisturizers containing niacinamide and glycerin significantly improved dry skin by providing a barrier against moisture loss, so that the skin remained hydrated. [60]

Panthenol (vitamin B5)

Percentage: 1 to 5% of the total formulation. Panthenol is very soluble in water, alcohol and glycerin, but not at all in oils. Thoroughly dissolve vitamin B5 powder in pure water or glycerin and filter it before you add it to any water-based skin formulations. Both glycerin and pure water are pH neutral.

VITAMIN E AND B SERUM

Ingredients:
- 2 ml (0.4 tsp) niacinamide powder
- 4 ml (0.8 tsp) panthenol powder
- 2 ml (0.4 tsp) goldenseal root powder
- 16 ml (approx. 3 tsp) pure rose flower water

---

60   *Two Randomized, Controlled, Comparative Studies of the Stratum Corneum Integrity Benefits of Two Cosmetic Niacinamide/Glycerin Body Moisturizers vs. Conventional Body Moisturizers. Jeremy C. Christman MS, Deborah K. Fix BS MBA, Sawanna C. Lucus BS, Debrah Watson BS, Emma Desmier BS, Rolanda J. Johnson Wilkerson PhD, Charles Fixler MD. Journal of Drugs in Dermatology VOLUME 11 • ISSUE 1 January 2012. Research sponsored by The Procter & Gamble Company, Cincinnati, OH and Private Practice, Cincinnati, OH*

- 16 ml (approx. 3 tsp) vegetable glycerin
- 10 ml (2 tsp) tocopheryl acetate
- 30 ml (6 tsp) cold-pressed wheat germ oil
- 40 ml (8 tsp) cold-pressed rice bran oil
- 40 ml (8 tsp) cold-pressed grapeseed oil
- 40 ml (8 tsp) cold-pressed sweet almond oil
- powdered milk (optional)

Instructions:
- Soak and stir the panthenol, niacinamide and goldenseal root powder in the rose flower water until they are completely dissolved.
- Strain the rose flower water through a fine wire strainer to remove any lumps.
- Add the glycerin and mix well.
- Now add the rest of the ingredients and whisk vigorously until all are thoroughly combined.
- If you wish to add texture to the serum, mix in some powdered milk, a little at a time, until the serum reaches your desired consistency.

Use and storage:
Follow the instructions for Home-made Retinol Serum. Shake well before using, as this mixture is likely to separate when left to stand.

HOME-MADE SKIN CARE: EXFOLIATING SCRUBS

HOME-MADE AHA (GLYCOLIC ACID) EXFOLIATING SCRUB

Glycolic acid is an alpha-hydroxy acid derived from sugar. The acid breaks the bonds between layers of skin cells, so that the dead skin cells of the outer layers can be scrubbed away. The younger skin beneath looks smoother and fresher.

Equipment:
- Small mixing bowl
- Spoon
- Cotton balls

Extras:
- Witch hazel or organic apple cider vinegar
- Basic skin cleanser
- Moisturizer
- Water

Ingredients for the peel:
2 tablespoons sugar
1 to 2 tablespoons plain yogurt

Ingredients for the rinse:
1 cup tea, cooled (green tea or chamomile)

Instructions:
- Combine the sugar with enough yogurt to make a creamy paste. The sugar will dissolve completely. This is the desired result: the undissolved grains act as an exfoliating scrub.
- Apply the sugar paste to your face. Avoid sensitive areas around your eyes, nostrils, and lip corners. Wait for about three minutes, then then splash on a few drops of water and use your fingertips to lightly massage the sugar paste over your skin.
- Rinse thoroughly with warm water. Use the tea as a final rinse to completely remove the sugar and yogurt paste and to soothe your skin.
- Massage the moisturizer into your skin while it is still damp.

CLEANSING SKIN EXFOLIANT

This skin-care recipe uses Fuller's Earth, which is available from cosmetic stores online. If you cannot buy Fuller's Earth, you can substitute Kaolin Clay, French Green Clay or Rhassoul Clay.

Ingredients:
- 3 parts wheat bran
- 1 part ground rice (rice flour)

- 1 part ground oats (oat flour)
- 1 part dried lemon peel
- 1 part organic cane sugar
- 1 part Fuller's Earth
- a few drops of vegetable glycerin

Instructions:
- Place all the dry ingredients (the first 6 ingredients) into a bowl and mix thoroughly.
- Pour mixture into an airtight container and keep it cool and dry until you are ready to use it.
- To prepare mixture for use, shake the container then place a small amount of it into a clean, dry ceramic bowl.
- Add enough water (a few drops) to make a thick paste. Stir with a spoon until water is absorbed evenly.
- Mix in a few drops of glycerin, according to your preference.

To use:
Apply lotion to damp skin and gently rub in a circular motion. Rinse it off with warm water and pat dry with a soft towel.

HOME-MADE SKIN CARE: SKIN PEELS

Before using peels
- Discontinue the use of any prescription formulations such as Retin-A for 5 days before and 10 days after glycolic acid and lactic acid peels.

- If you are using chemical peels for the first time, use the lowest concentration peel and gradually move up to stronger peels as your skin gets used to them.
- Lighter peels can be safely done every two weeks.
- Two days before you use the peel, start cleansing your skin with a soap-free cleanser. The peel will penetrate your skin better, and all acid peels work best when the skin is not too alkaline.
- Have on hand your neutralizer, moisturizer and sunscreen for post-peel treatment.
- Do a spot test on a small patch of your skin, 24 hours before you give yourself a full-face chemical peel. to find out how your skin will react.
- People who are allergic to aspirin should not use peels containing BHA.
- AHA and BHA peels can cause temporary skin irritation and redness. If symptoms persist or get worse, stop using the peel immediately.
- Skin peels will probably make your skin quite photosensitive, so make sure you wear a good sunscreen if you go outdoors.

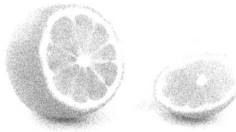

HOME-MADE AHA (CITRIC & LACTIC ACID) FACIAL PEEL

Lemon juice is an alpha hydroxy acid that contains vitamin C. It acts as a peel and is also an excellent antioxidant and skin food.

Equipment:
- Small bowl
- Spoon
- Shallow dish
- Cotton balls

Extras:
- Witch hazel or organic apple cider vinegar
- Basic skin cleanser
- Moisturizer
- Sunscreen

Ingredients:
1-½ tablespoons full-fat milk
1-2 tsp freshly squeezed lemon juice
1 small slice of lemon

Instructions:
- In a small ceramic or glass bowl, combine the lemon juice and milk.
- Add the lemon slice.
- Allow the bowl to stand, at room temperature, for four hours. During this time the mixture will curdle; it is normal for it to do so.

To use:
- Wash your face, pat it dry and swab it with witch hazel or organic apple cider vinegar.
- After the witch hazel dries, apply the peel mixture. Avoid sensitive areas around your eyes, nostrils, and lip corners.
- Leave it on for one minute if using it for the first time - longer if your skin is already used to it.
- Wash it off completely with your basic skin cleanser.
- Pat your face dry, then moisturize.

HOME-MADE BHA (SALICYLIC ACID) FACIAL PEEL

Salicylic acid, derived from willow bark, is used in aspirin. People who are allergic to aspirin should not use this peel.

Equipment:
- Small bowl
- Spoon
- Shallow dish
- Cotton balls

Extras:
- Witch hazel or organic apple cider vinegar
- Basic skin cleanser
- Moisturizer

Ingredients:
1 tablespoon baking soda
1 cup water
12 uncoated aspirin pills (generic brands are fine)
Juice of 1 lemon

Instructions:
- Place the baking soda and water into the bowl and stir until the baking soda is thoroughly dissolved. Set aside.
- Put the aspirin pills in the shallow dish crush them into a powder with the back of a spoon.
- Sprinkle the lemon juice over the powder, a few drops at a time, mixing the aspirin into a thin paste. If necessary, add more lemon juice.

To use:
- Wash your face, pat it dry and swab it with witch hazel or organic apple cider vinegar.
- After the witch hazel dries, apply the lemon-and-aspirin mixture. Avoid sensitive areas around your eyes, nostrils, and lip corners.
- Leave it on for one minute if using it for the first time - longer if your skin is already used to it.
- Wipe off the peel with cotton balls soaked in the baking soda neutralizer.
- Wash off the baking soda with your basic skin cleanser.
- Pat your face dry, then moisturize.

HOME-MADE SKIN CARE:
PORE REFINING TREATMENTS

Large pores are typically caused by excessively oily skin, sun-damaged skin, or — in many cases — decreased skin elasticity due to the natural aging process.

Although there is no way to permanently get rid of enlarged facial pores, there are some treatments that you can use on a daily or weekly basis, either at home or in a clinic or salon, to reduce their appearance.

Cleansing, exfoliating and peeling the skin will greatly improve the appearance of pores, as will the correct removal of blackheads and whiteheads. See the section on extraction of comedones, page 56.

However, if you wish to minimize the appearance of pores still further, you can try using a pore refining mask.

The following recipe is for a mask that should be applied to the skin as soon as it is made.

Discard any leftovers, and make a new batch each time you use it. It can be used once a day, if needed, but no oftener.

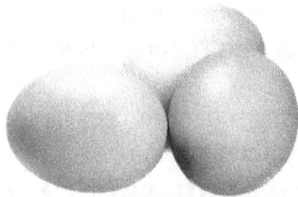

CUCUMBER AND EGG PORE REFINING MASK

Egg yolk oil (which is derived from the yolk of chicken eggs) is rich in omega-3 fatty acids and omega-6 fatty acids. It closely resembles the lipid profile of human skin. Applying raw egg white to the skin can have a temporary tightening effect. Pastured eggs contain far more nutrients than cage eggs. Choose free-range eggs if pastured eggs are unavailable.

Equipment:
- Bowl
- Wire whisk
- Blender or food processor
- Small mixing bowl

Ingredients:
- 2 large pastured eggs
- 2 tablespoons all-purpose (plain) flour
- 1 small cucumber
- Luke-warm water

Instructions:
- Crack the eggs into the bowl and whisk them thoroughly.
- Add flour and continue whisking until the flour has blended completely and the mixture is smooth.
- Set it aside to thicken.
- Peel and roughly chop the cucumber, then put it in the blender.
- Purée the cucumber until it is smooth.
- Add the egg and flour mixture to the puréed cucumber.
- Process again on medium speed until all the ingredients are combined.

To Use:
- Gently wash and dry your face.
- Using clean hand or cotton balls, apply the mixture directly to the face.
- Leave it on for ten minutes before rinsing thoroughly with luke-warm water.

- Pat your face dry, then moisturize.

SIMPLE LEMON JUICE AND EGG PORE REFINING TREATMENT

This treatment not only helps to temporarily refine pores, it also acts as a peel and exfoliant.

Equipment:
- Soft, clean toothbrush
- Small mixing bowl

Ingredients:
- 1 pastured or free-range egg
- Juice of half a lemon
- Lukewarm water

Instructions:

Separate the egg white from the yolk.

Place the egg white into the small mixing bowl.

Mix in a few drops of lemon juice and stir until the mixture froths.

To use:
- Dip the toothbrush into the bowl and use it to massage the mixture onto the skin.
- Leave the mixture on your skin for about five minutes before rinsing it off with lukewarm water.
- Pat your face dry, then moisturize.

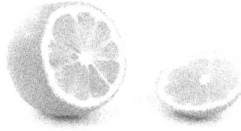

HOME-MADE SKIN CARE: SKIN LIGHTENING TREATMENTS

Large numbers of natural extracts have been scientifically shown to lighten discoloration or pigmentation of the skin. See "Skin Therapy: skin lightening creams" on page 233.

SIMPLE LEMON JUICE SKIN LIGHTENER

Ascorbic acid (vitamin C) which is abundant in lemon juice, is considered to be a skin whitening agent. Dip a cotton ball in freshly squeezed lemon juice and apply it to the discolored patches of your skin. Leave it to dry for about an hour, then wash it off with lukewarm water. Pat your skin dry and apply moisturizer. Do not use this treatment more than once every 24 hours.

LEMON JUICE AND TURMERIC SKIN LIGHTENER

Mix three teaspoons of lemon juice and one teaspoon of turmeric powder to make a paste. Apply the paste to the discolored areas of skin and leave it on for half an hour. Pat your skin dry and apply moisturizer. Do not use this treatment more than once every 24 hours.

SIMPLE ALOE VERA SKIN LIGHTENER

Aloe vera can be grown outdoors in temperate to warm climates. Pick some leaves of aloe vera then snip through the skin of the leaves with a sharp pair of scissors. Squeeze out the content, which are thick and jelly-like. With clean hands or cotton balls, apply this gel directly to the discolored skin. Leave it on for about half an hour before rinsing it off with luke-warm water. Repeat daily.

HOME-MADE SKIN CARE: SUNSCREENS

All commercially available sunscreens should provide adequate protection from the sun's harmful ultraviolet rays (UVA and UVB).

There are two types of sunscreens—chemical and physical. Chemical sunscreens absorbs UV rays, while physical sunscreens reflects the damaging wavelengths away from the skin.

Physical sunblocks

The two most common physical sunblocks are zinc oxide and titanium dioxide. Both of them give broad-spectrum UVA and UVB protection. They rarely cause skin irritation and thus are useful for children and people with sensitive skin.

Some people do not like using them, because their ray-reflecting action makes the skin appear paler.

Chemical sunblocks

Most chemical sunscreen formulations only block a small section of the UV wavelength spectrum. This means that manufacturers have to include several chemical ingredients, with each one blocking a different section of UV light.

Most chemicals used in sunscreen products can only block out rays in the UVB section. Very few can block UVA rays.

Many sunscreen products contain chemicals that have not been around for long enough to be proved safe for long-term human use. For example, the inclusion of microfine or nano-particle titanium dioxide as an ingredient has no long-term safety data.

Zinc oxide

Safe and natural sunscreens use zinc oxide as their active ingredient and contain no nano-particles. They provide broad-spectrum protection from UVA and UVB rays and are designed to sit on top of the skin and reflect rays. They require less frequent re-application than absorbable sunscreens do. They can also clog your pores however, and must be thoroughly washed off when no longer needed.

Other natural ingredients

Coconut oil, sesame oil, olive oil vitamin E and zinc all provide some (limited) protection from ultraviolet (UV) light. Studies show that sesame oil resists 30% of UV rays while coconut and olive oils block out about 20% of UV rays. Vitamin E can also absorb the energy from UV rays.

Turmeric, coffee and cocoa can be used in zinc oxide sunscreens to improve the color and offset zinc's whiteness.

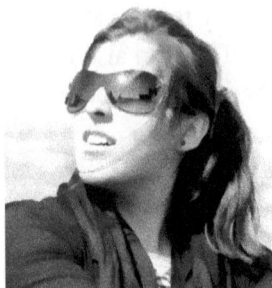

BASIC HOME-MADE SUNSCREEN

Xanthan gum is essential in this recipe. It thickens the lotion so that is becomes easier to apply. It also stabilizes the emulsion and prevents it from separating into liquids and solids, while keeping the zinc oxide in suspension. Xanthan gum is available from health food stores and online.

To prolong shelf life use ingredients that are as fresh as possible, and sterilize/sanitize all your tools beforehand (for example, using boiling water or Milton® Sterilizing Fluid),

Make small batches at a time so that you can use it all up while it is still fresh.

Some people like to add a preservative such as Liquid Germall® Plus. Three drops should be enough to keep one batch fresher for longer.

Ingredients:

Water mixture:
- ⅓ cup witch hazel (or 5 tbsp if you do not use coffee)
- 2 tsp fresh coffee grounds (optional)

Oil mixture:
- 1 tbsp coconut oil
- 1 ¼ tsp emulsifying wax
- ½ tsp extra virgin olive oil

- ½ tsp sesame oil
- 2 tsp cocoa powder (optional)

Powder mixture:
- 1 to 2 tbsp non-nano-particulated zinc oxide (available from soap-making suppliers, drugstores/pharmacies or online)
- 1 small pinch xanthan gum
- ½ tsp powdered turmeric, for a color tint (optional)

Extras:
- ¼ tsp liquid vitamin E
- ¼ tsp rose flower water

Instructions:
- In a double boiler slowly heat the oil mix till all ingredients are melted and well blended.
- In a separate container warm the witch hazel with the coffee.
- Meanwhile sift the powder mix together.
- Remove the witch hazel mix from heat. If you used coffee pass the liquid through a paper filter and add an extra tablespoon of witch hazel.
- Slowly drip the oil mix into the witch hazel, blending with a fork, whisk or hand-held stick mixer till all the oil is mixed in and emulsified.
- Blend in the powder mix, then the vitamin E and rose flower water.
- Pour into a sterilized, dry jar or other container with a lid. Attach a label with the name of the formulation and the date on which it was made.

To use:
Zinc oxide sunscreen cream works immediately. Dip into the jar with clean fingers and apply it generously before you go outdoors, even when the day is overcast. Sunscreen should be reapplied if it has

been rubbed off - for example after you go swimming or after you've been sweating.

HOME-MADE TEMPORARY SKIN-TIGHTENING MASKS

Applying egg whites to your skin and allowing them to dry can give the effect of skin tightening, although this is only temporary. Usually, the effect only lasts for about an hour after the mask has been rinsed off.

There is, nonetheless, an added benefit of egg white masks. When you use egg whites as a carrier base and mix in other ingredients, you can deliver the added benefits of those ingredients to your skin.

Egg white masks may also help oily skin. As the egg whites dry and tighten, skin oils are pulled into it.

Egg white masks are safe enough to be used several times a week without causing any skin damage whatsoever. Of course we recommend that you avoid egg as an ingredient in any skincare product if you have an egg allergy. Different people react to different substances, so we also recommend that if you are adding other ingredients to your egg white mask, you first test the mask by applying a little of it on the inside of your elbow. If your skin does not have any adverse reactions, go ahead and use the formulation on your face.

EGG WHITE SKIN TIGHTENING MASK

Ingredients:
1 pastured or free-range egg
1 tsp cornstarch (cornflour)

Instructions:
Separate the egg white from the yolk.[61]

Place the egg white and the cornstarch in a small bowl and whisk thoroughly with a fork, until all lumps have disappeared.

---

61   *You could eat the leftover yolks, or make a hair mask with them by mixing them with 1 tablespoon of olive oil. Apply hair mask to wet hair, cover with a shower cap and leave for 20 minutes. Rinse off with cool water.*

To use:

Apply the egg white mixture directly to your face, using your fingers. Wait until it dries (around 20 minutes), then rinse it off with lukewarm water.

We recommend that you lie on your back while the mask is drying.

To the basic egg white mixture you can add ingredients such as:
- Almond oil (for dry skin)
- Avocado
- Cabbage leaves
- Fullers' Earth
- Glycerin (for dry skin)
- Grated potato or apple
- Honey
- Rice flour
- Sugar
- Yoghurt

ABOUT FULLER'S EARTH

'Fuller's Earth is any clay material that has the capability to decolorize oil or other liquids without chemical treatment. Fuller's Earth typically consists of palygorskite (attapulgite) or bentonite clay. Modern uses of Fuller's Earth include absorbents for oil, grease, and animal waste and as a carrier for pesticides and fertilizers. Minor uses include filtering, clarifying, and decolorizing; and as filler in paint, plaster, adhesives, and pharmaceuticals.

'The name reflects the historic use of the material for cleaning or "fulling" wool by textile workers called "fullers". In past centuries, fullers kneaded Fuller's Earth and water into woolen cloth to absorb lanolin, oils, and other greasy impurities as part of the cloth finishing process. Fuller's Earth is also sometimes referred to as 'bleaching clay', probably because fulling whitened the cloth.

'In addition to its original use in the fulling of raw fibers, Fuller's Earth is now utilized in a number of industries. Most important applications make use of the minerals' natural absorbent properties in products sold as absorbents or filters.

'Medicine: Fuller's Earth is used (with activated charcoal) in the treatment of paraquat poisoning to prevent the progression to pulmonary fibrosis.

'Decontamination: Fuller's Earth is used by military and civil emergency service personnel to decontaminate the clothing and equipment of servicemen and CBRN (Chemical Biological Radiological Nuclear) responders who have been contaminated with chemical agents.

'Personal care: Fuller's Earth has been used in the Indian subcontinent as a face pack and cleanser for thousands of years, and is known as also known as 'Multani Mitti Clay' – that is, mud from Multan. It has been used as an ingredient in powdered, "dry" shampoos, and is an important ingredient in many face packs. Fuller's Earth was also sold in pharmacies until recently for compressing pills and cleaning hats and fabrics.

'Cleaning Agent: In the Indian subcontinent, it has been used for centuries to clean marble. As a good absorbent, it removes the surface of dust, dirt, impurities and stains and replenishes the shine of the marble. It has been used numerous times to clean one of the most spectacular buildings in the white marble, that of the Taj Mahal, in Agra, India with positive results.'[62]

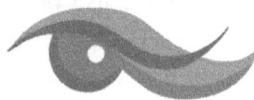

---

62   Fuller's Earth. Wikipedia, the free encyclopedia. Article retrieved 28.7.14

INDEX

F

I

J

K

L

M

S

T

TCA peel. 81
tear troughs 29, 110, 160, 161
teeth 24, 106, 175
temporary eyebrow tinting 123
thinning skin 26, 46, 228
threading 121, 171, 211
thread lift 88, 140
tinting/dyeing 122
tips for eyebrow grooming 124
topical wrinkle treatments 37
traditional facelift 131
treatments for skin discoloration 64
tretinoin 63, 70
trichloroacetic acid 63, 81, 197
trichotillomania 40
trichotillosis 40
'turkey' neck 26
Types of Acne Scars 48
  boxcar scars 49
  ice pick scars 48
  rolling scars 50
types of eczema 74
types of lasers 206
hypertrophic or keloid scars 50

U

ultrasound skin therapy 96
ultraviolet light. 59
ultraviolet radiation therapy 75, 77, 247
uneven skin tone 26, 46
unwanted tattoos 102
urea 68, 76, 77, 189

V

varicose veins 98
vitamin A serum 70
vitamin C serum 38, 45, 62, 69, 186, 272, 274
vitiligo 60

W

About the author:

Elizabeth Reed is a university graduate and author with an interest in researching the 'science of beauty'. She spent a year writing the 'Beauty' series, examining studies from across the globe. She lives with her husband in Australia, and is the mother of three children.

Also from Leaves of Gold Press:

THE NEW BESTSELLER

IS
FOOD
MAKING YOU
SICK?

With more than 100 recipes

The
Strictly Low Histamine Diet

ECZEMA sleep disorders REFLUX *nausea* anxiety
SINUSITIS stomach PAIN *fuzzy* thinking *itching*
joint pain irritability *hives* HEADACHES bowel DISEASE
asthma inflammation hayfever DIZZINESS diarrhea *migraines*

and more . . .

James L. Gibb

IS FOOD MAKING YOU SICK?

THE STRICTLY LOW HISTAMINE DIET

By James L. Gibb

People all over the world suffer from histamine intolerance without being aware of it.

The symptoms are many and widely varied, often resembling food allergies or other diseases. They can affect the digestive system, the respiratory system, the skin and many other parts of the body. These problems may endure throughout our entire lives if we continue to consume large amounts of histamine.

Histamine is colorless, odorless and tasteless - undetectable except by scientific analysis, and yet crucial to our well-being.

Individual histamine tolerance thresholds vary greatly. A range of circumstances including our genes, our environment, our diet and stress, cause our bodies' histamine levels to rise.

If they rise faster than our bodies can break them down, we experience the excessive inflammation brought on by histamine intolerance, or HIT.

The good news is, if we can understand what is happening and why, we can treat or prevent this widely unrecognized but very real condition.

Notes

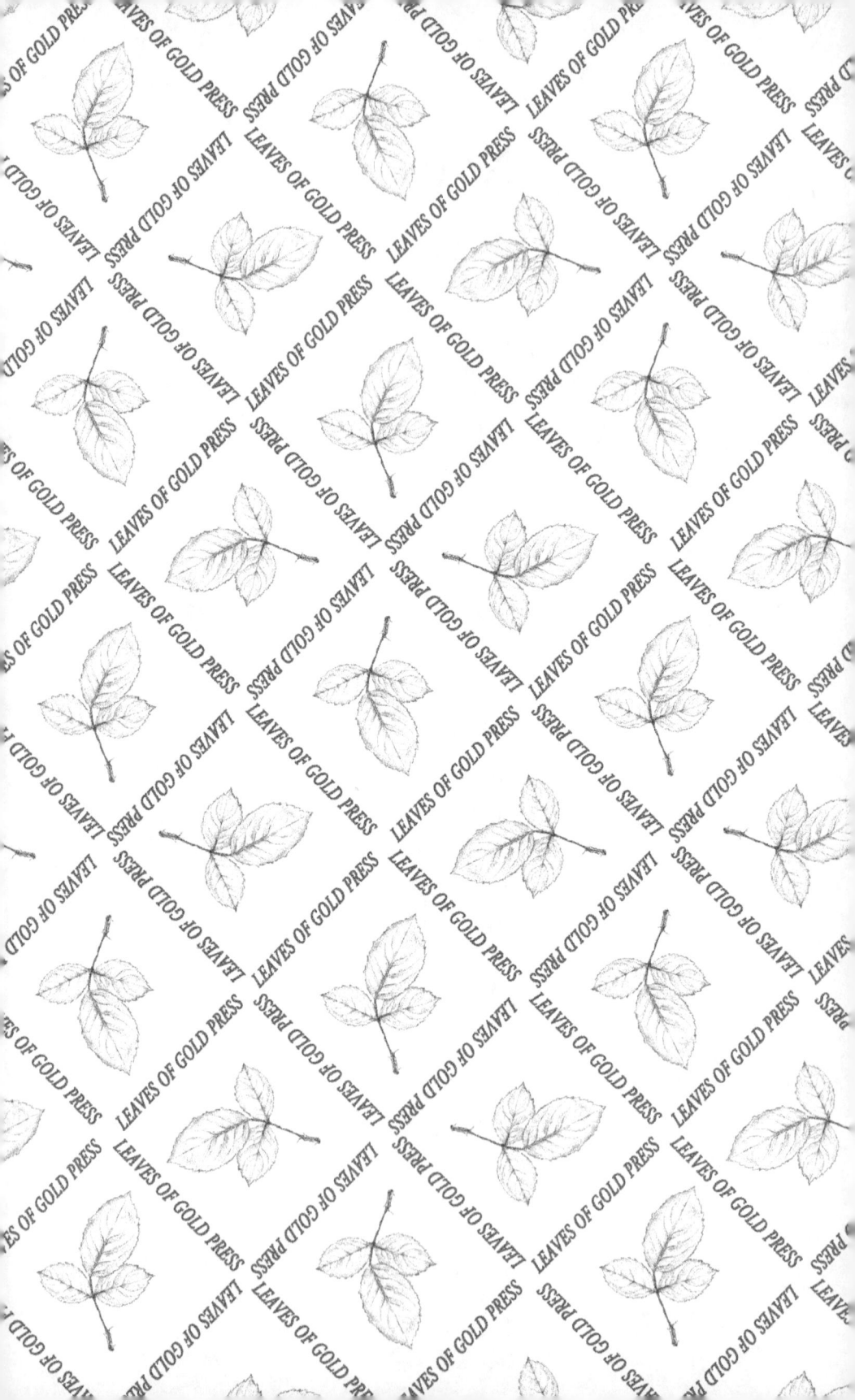

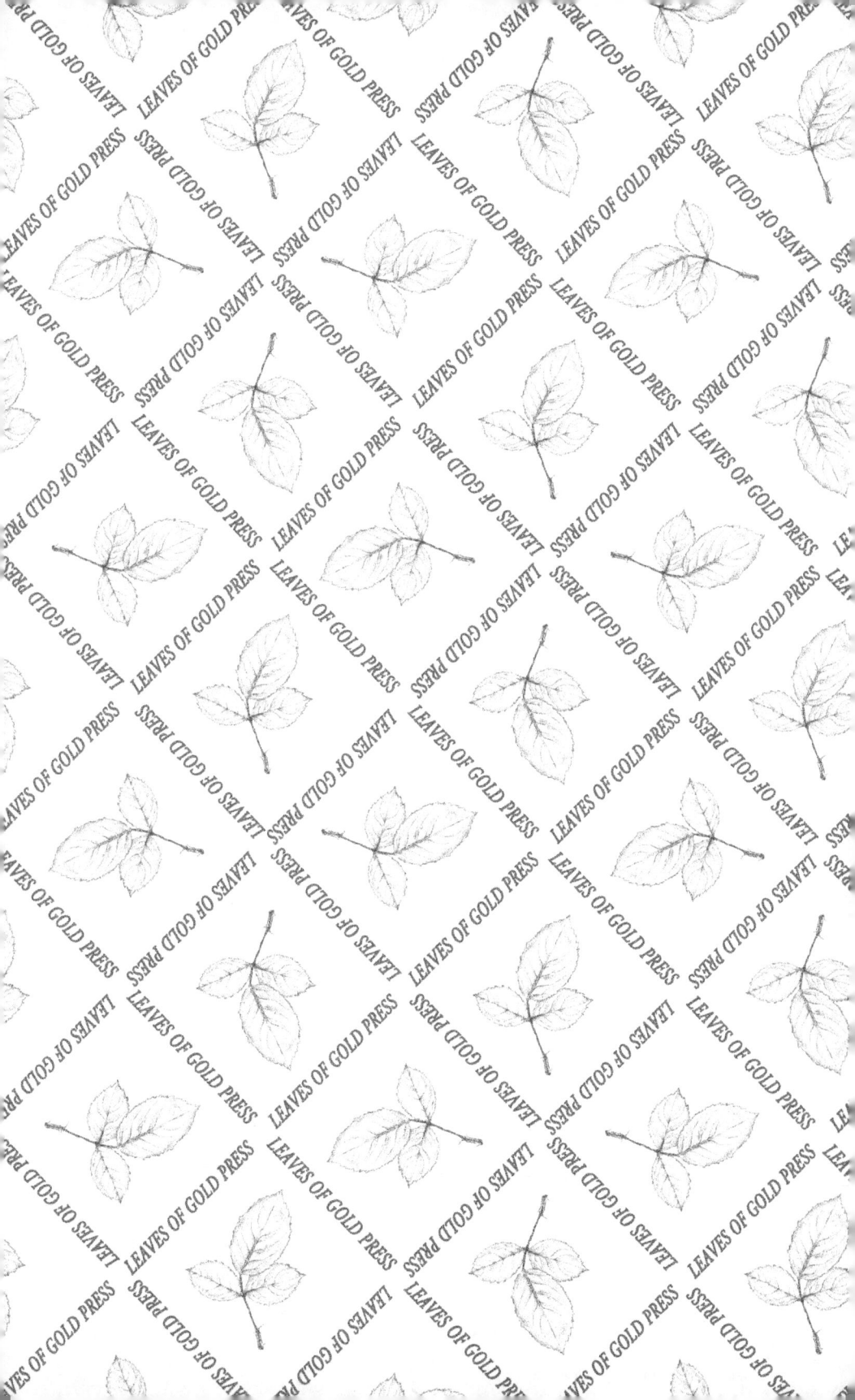